T0332241

Mathematical Modeling of Virus Infection

ODE/PDE Analysis in R

Mathematical Modeling of Virus Infection

ODE/PDE Analysis in R

William E Schiesser

Lehigh University, USA

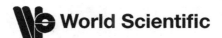 World Scientific

NEW JERSEY · LONDON · SINGAPORE · BEIJING · SHANGHAI · HONG KONG · TAIPEI · CHENNAI · TOKYO

Published by

World Scientific Publishing Co. Pte. Ltd.

5 Toh Tuck Link, Singapore 596224

USA office: 27 Warren Street, Suite 401-402, Hackensack, NJ 07601

UK office: 57 Shelton Street, Covent Garden, London WC2H 9HE

British Library Cataloguing-in-Publication Data
A catalogue record for this book is available from the British Library.

MATHEMATICAL MODELING OF VIRUS INFECTION
ODE/PDE Analysis in R

ISBN 978-981-123-663-1 (hardcover)
ISBN 978-981-123-664-8 (ebook for institutions)
ISBN 978-981-123-665-5 (ebook for individuals)

For any available supplementary material, please visit
https://www.worldscientific.com/worldscibooks/10.1142/12267#t=suppl

Typeset by Stallion Press
Email: enquiries@stallionpress.com

Printed in Singapore

Contents

Preface

This book details two models pertaining to the dynamics of infection from a virus:

(1) Lung/respiratory system model

The lung/respiratory system model gives the spatiotemporal distribution of four viral-related proteins:

> Virus population density along the lung air passage.

> Host cell primary infection protein (viral genetic material (VGM)) concentration.

> Host cell secondary infection protein (VGM) concentration.

> Air stream virion population density

The spatiotemporal distribution of the four component proteins is computed as the solution of a system of partial differential equations (PDEs). The independent variables are position along the lung (air passage) and time. The basic algorithm is the method of lines (MOL), a general numerical method for PDEs. The programming is in R, a quality, open-source scientific computing system.

The model is executed for a single inhalation, and a series of inhalation/exhalation cycles. For the latter, the progression of the viral infection into the lung is a principal result.

(2) SVIR model

The SVIR (**S**usceptible-**V**accinated-**I**nfected-**R**ecovered) model is formulated as a system of ordinary differential equations (ODEs) in time, then extended to a system of partial differential equations (PDEs) to account for spatial effects (spatiotemporal modeling).

The PDE model is stated for a polar (radial) domain that can represent a geographical region. The dispersion of the virus within this region is modeled as a diffusion process so that the PDEs are diffusion equations in time and space, t and r. The output from the ODE model, $S(t)$, $V(t)$, $I(t)$, $R(t)$ is extended in the PDE model to $S(r,t)$, $V(r,t)$, $I(r,t)$, $R(r,t)$. Boundary conditions (BCs) for the PDE model include the transfer of susceptible, vaccinated, infected and recovered populations, $S(r,t)$, $V(r,t)$, $I(r,t)$, $R(r,t)$ across the radial domain outer boundary.

A principal output from the ODE/PDE models is the level of vaccinations, $V(t)$, $V(r,t)$ and infections, $I(t)$, $I(r,t)$. For the latter, the efficacy of the vaccine is a parameter that can be varied in a computer-based analysis of a vaccine therapy.

The programming is in R, with the PDE model integrated (solved) by the MOL. The R routines are available from a download link so that the example models can be executed without having to first study numerical methods and computer coding. The routines can then be applied to variations and extensions of the ODE/PDE models, such as changes in the parameters and the form of the model equations.

The author would welcome comments/suggestions concerning this approach to the analysis of virus infection dynamics (directed to wes1@lehigh.edu).

W. E. Schiesser
Bethlehem, PA, USA

Chapter 1

Lung/Respiratory System Model Formulation

(1) Introduction

Viral invasion of the lung/respiratory system is a major health problem as reflected in SARS, MERS and COVID-19. The development and implementaion of a mathematical model for viral lung invasion and infection is presented in this chapter. The solution of the model gives the spatiotemporal distribution of four viral-related proteins, as listed in Table 1.1.

$u_1(z,t)$ virus population density along the lung air passage

$u_2(z,t)$ host cell primary infection protein (viral genetic material (VGM)) concentration

$u_3(z,t)$ host cell secondary infection protein (VGM) concentration

$u_4(z,t)$ air stream virion population density

z position along the lung (air passage)

t time

Table 1.1: PDE model variables

(1.1) PDE model formulation

The spatiotemporal evolution of $u_1(z,t), u_2(z,t), u_3(z,t), u_4(z,t)$ is defined by the PDE model developed next. Of particular interest is:

(1) Invasion of the virus from the air to lung host cells, $u_1(z,t)$ to $u_2(z,t)$.
(2) Production of additional viral genetic material (VGM) in the host cells, possibly with mutation of the DNA/RNA. $u_2(z,t)$ to $u_3(z,t)$.
(3) Net movement of the VGM from the host cells to the air which is then discharged from the lungs, $u_3(z,t)$ to $u_4(z,t)$.

Each of the four dependent variables listed in Table 1.1 is defined by a PDE.

The PDE for $u_1(z,t)$ follows as eq. (1.1-1).

$$\frac{\partial u_1(z,t)}{\partial t} = -v_1(t)\frac{\partial u_1(z,t)}{\partial z} + k_{m12}\left(\frac{1}{k_{e12}}u_2(z,t) - u_1(z,t)\right)$$

$$(1.1\text{-}1)$$

where

$v_1(t)$	velocity of air flow through the lung
	$v_1(t) \geq 0$, inhalation
	$v_1(t) < 0$, exhalation

k_{m12}	mass transfer coefficient defining the flux of virus from the air stream to the host cell population

$k_{e12} = \dfrac{u_2(z,t)}{u_1(z,t)}$	equilibrium constant relating $u_2(z,t)$ to $u_1(z,t)$ at equilibtium

Table 1.2a: Parameters of eq. (1.1-1)

The terms in eq. (1.1-1) constitute a virus population balance for an incremental volume of the lung of length Δz, that is, $\epsilon A_c \Delta z$, where A_c is the effective lung cross sectional area and ϵ is the fractional volume of the air passage. As explained in the derivation of eq. (1.1-1) in chapter Appendix A1, the limit $\Delta z \to 0$ gives the PDE, eq. (1.1-1).

The individual terms in eq. (1.1-1) are explained next.

- $\dfrac{\partial u_1(z,t)}{\partial t}$: Time rate of change of the virus population in the incremental volume.
- $-v_1(t)\dfrac{\partial u_1(z,t)}{\partial z}$: Net convection of the virus into or out of the incremental volume.
- $k_{m12}(\dfrac{1}{k_{e12}}u_2(z,t) - u_1(z,t))$: Rate of mass transfer of the virus from the air to host cells.

The PDE for $u_2(z,t)$ follows as eq. (1.1-2).

$$\frac{\partial u_2(z,t)}{\partial t} = -k_{m12}(u_2(z,t) - k_{e12}u_1(z,t)) - r_2 u_2(z,t)^{n_2} \quad (1.1\text{-}2)$$

where

r_2	rate constant for conversion of primary protein in the host cells to secondary protein
n_2	order for conversion of primary protein in the host cells to secondary protein

Table 1.2b: Parameters of eq. (1.1-2)

The terms in eq. (1.1-2) constitute a primary protein balance for an incremental volume of the lung of length Δz, that is, $(1 - \epsilon)A_c \Delta z$. As explained in the derivation of eq. (1.1-2) in chapter Appendix A1, the limit $\Delta z \to 0$ gives the PDE, eq. (1.1-2).

The individual terms in eq. (1.1-2) are explained next.

- $\dfrac{\partial u_2(z,t)}{\partial t}$: Time rate of change of the primary protein (DNA, RNA) in the incremental volume.
- $-k_{m12}(u_2(z,t) - k_{e12}u_1(z,t))$: Rate of mass transfer of the virus from the air to host cells.
- $-r_2 u_2(z,t)^{n_2}$: Volumetric rate of production of a secondary protein (DNA, RNA) in the host cells.

The PDE for $u_3(z,t)$ follows as eq. (1.1-3).

$$\frac{\partial u_3(z,t)}{\partial t} = -k_{m34}(u_3(z,t) - \frac{1}{k_{e34}}u_4(z,t)) + r_2 u_2(z,t)^{n_2} \qquad (1.1\text{-}3)$$

where

k_{m34}	mass transfer coefficient defining the flux of the secondary protein from the host cells to the air stream
$k_{e34} = \dfrac{u_4(z,t)}{u_3(z,t)}$	equilibrium constant relating $u_4(z,t)$ to $u_3(z,t)$ at equilibrium

Table 1.2c: Parameters of eq. (1.1-3)

The terms in eq. (1.1-3) constitute a secondary protein balance for an incremental volume of the lung of length Δz, that is, $(1 - \epsilon)A_c \Delta z$. As explained in the derivation of eq. (1.1-3) in chapter Appendix A1, the limit $\Delta z \to 0$ gives the PDE, eq. (1.1-3).

The individual terms in eq. (1.1-3) are explained next.

- $\dfrac{\partial u_3(z,t)}{\partial t}$: Time rate of change of the secondary protein (DNA, RNA) in the incremental volume.
- $-k_{m34}(u_3(z,t) - \dfrac{1}{k_{e34}}u_4(z,t))$: mass transfer of the secondary protein from the host cells to the air stream.

- $r_2 u_2(z,t)^{n_2}$: Volumetric rate of production of a secondary protein (DNA, RNA) in the host cells.

The PDE for $u_4(z,t)$ follows as eq. (1.1-4)[1].

$$\frac{\partial u_4(z,t)}{\partial t} = -v_1(t)\frac{\partial u_4(z,t)}{\partial z} + k_{m34}(k_{e34}u_3(z,t) - u_4(z,t))$$

(1.1-4)

The parameters in eq. (1.1-4) are explained in Tables 1.2.

The terms in eq. (1.1-4) constitute a virion population balance for an incremental volume of the lung of length Δz, that is, $\epsilon A_c \Delta z$. As explained in the derivation of eq. (1.1-4) in chapter Appendix A1, the limit $\Delta z \to 0$ gives the PDE, eq. (1.1-4).

The individual terms in eq. (1.1-4) are explained next.

- $\dfrac{\partial u_4(z,t)}{\partial t}$: Time rate of change of the virion population in the incremental volume.
- $-v_1(t)\dfrac{\partial u_4(z,t)}{\partial z}$: Net convection of the virions into or out of the incremental volume.
- $k_{m34}(k_{e34}u_3(z,t) - u_4(z,t))$: Rate of mass transfer of the secondary protein from the host cells to the air stream (to produce virions).

Eqs. (1.1) are first order in t and each requires one initial condition (IC).

$$u_1(x, t = 0) = u_{10}(z) \qquad\qquad (1.2\text{-}1)$$

$$u_2(x, t = 0) = u_{20}(z) \qquad\qquad (1.2\text{-}2)$$

---

[1]The secondary protein particles that enter the air stream are termed *virions*, that is, viruses that can invade other normal (healthy) cells which is the mechanism for the spread of the virus.

$$u_3(x, t = 0) = u_{30}(z) \qquad (1.2\text{-}3)$$

$$u_4(x, t = 0) = u_{40}(z) \qquad (1.2\text{-}4)$$

Eqs. (1.1-1,4) are first order in z and each requires one boundary condition (BC).

For $v_1(t) > 0$,

$$u_1(x = 0, t) = u_{1b}(t) \qquad (1.3\text{-}1)$$

$$u_4(x = 0, t) = u_{4b}(t) \qquad (1.3\text{-}2)$$

where $u_{1b}(t), u_{4b}(t)$ are functions to be specified.

For $v_1(t) < 0$, eqs. (1.1-1,4) with no convection are used as BCs.

$$\frac{\partial u_1(z = z_u, t)}{\partial t} = k_{12} \left(\frac{1}{k_{e12}} u_2(z = z_u, t) - u_1(z = z_u, t) \right)$$
$$(1.3\text{-}3)$$

$$\frac{\partial u_4(z = z_u, t)}{\partial t} = k_{34}(k_{e34} u_3(z = z_u, t) - u_4(z = z_u, t)) \qquad (1.3\text{-}4)$$

where z_u is the axial length of the lung air passage way ($z_u = 20$ cm defined for the spatial grid in Listing 2.1).

Eqs. (1.1), (1.2), (1.3) constitute the four PDE model for the lung/respiratory system.

(1.2) Summary and conclusions

The 4×4 (four equations in four unknowns) PDE model for the lung/respiratory system has been developed and explained. In general, the invasion of the virus into the lung tissue and the production of virions that can further infect lung tissue is a principal output of the PDE model.

The implementation of the model is discussed in Chapter 2.

Appendix A1: Derivation of the four PDE model

The derivation of the $u_1(z,t)$ PDE, eq. (1.1-1), is based on a virus population balance for an incremental volume $\epsilon A_c \Delta z$.

$$\epsilon A_c \Delta z \frac{\partial u_1(z,t)}{\partial t} =$$

$$v_1(z,t)\epsilon A_c u_1(z,t)|_{z-\Delta z} - v_1(z,t)\epsilon A_c u_1(z,t)|_z$$

$$+\epsilon A_c \Delta z k_{m12}(\frac{1}{k_{e12}}u_2(z,t) - u_1(z,t)) \tag{A1.1}$$

An explanation of the terms in eq. (A1.1) follows.

- $\epsilon A_c \Delta z \dfrac{\partial u_1(z,t)}{\partial t}$: Change in the virus population with t.
  With subscripts l, a, c for lung, air space, cells (tissue), $\epsilon = \dfrac{cm_a^3}{cm_l^3}$, $k_{m12} = \dfrac{1}{sec}$, $k_{e12} = \dfrac{\dfrac{cm_c^3}{virus\ population}}{cm_a^3}$

  the units of the term are:

$$(\frac{cm_a^3}{cm_l^3})(cm_l^2)(cm_l)\left(\frac{virus\ population}{cm_a^3 - sec}\right) = \frac{virus\ population}{sec}$$

In summary, the net units are $\dfrac{virus\ population}{sec}$.

- $v_1(z,t)\epsilon A_c u_1(z,t)|_{z-\Delta z}$: Virus entering the incremental volume at $z - \Delta z$. The units of the term are:

$$(\frac{cm_l}{sec})(\frac{cm_a^3}{cm_l^3})(cm_l^2)\left(\frac{virus\ population}{cm_a^3}\right) = \frac{virus\ population}{sec}$$

The convective term at z has the same units as the preceding $\dfrac{\partial u_1(z,t)}{\partial t}$ term.

- $\epsilon A_c \Delta z k_{m12}(\frac{1}{k_{e12}}u_2(z,t) - u_1(z,t))$: Rate of transfer of virus to host cells. The units of the term are:

$$\frac{cm_a^3}{cm_l^3}(cm_l^2)(cm_l)\frac{1}{sec}\left(\frac{\dfrac{virus\ population}{cm_a^3}}{\dfrac{primary\ protein\ concentration}{cm_c^3}}\right.$$

$$\left.\frac{primary\ protein\ concentration}{cm_c^3} - \frac{virus\ population}{cm_a^3}\right) =$$

$$\frac{virus\ population}{sec}$$

The mass transfer term, $k_{m12}(\frac{1}{k_{e12}}u_2(z,t) - u_1(z,t))$, involves the difference of the primary protein concentration (in the cells) and the virus population (in the air passage).

Minor rearrangement of eq. (A1.1) gives

$$\frac{\partial u_1(z,t)}{\partial t} =$$

$$-\left(\frac{v_1(z,t)u_1(z,t)|_z - v_1(z,t)u_1(z,t)|_{z-\Delta z}}{\Delta z}\right)$$

$$+k_{m12}(\frac{1}{k_{e12}}u_2(z,t) - u_1(z,t)) \qquad (A1.2)$$

In the limit $\Delta z \to 0$, eq. (A1.2) is

$$\frac{\partial u_1(z,t)}{\partial t} = -\left(\frac{\partial v_1(z,t)u_1(z,t)}{\partial z}\right) + k_{m12}(\frac{1}{k_{e12}}u_2(z,t) - u_1(z,t))$$
$$(A1.3)$$

For $v_1(z,t) = v_1(t)$, eq. (A1.3) is eq. (1.1-1).

The derivation of the $u_2(z,t)$ PDE, eq. (1.1-2), is based on a primary protein balance for an incremental volume $(1-\epsilon)A_c\Delta z$.

$$(1-\epsilon)A_c\Delta z\frac{\partial u_2(z,t)}{\partial t} =$$

$$-(1-\epsilon)A_c\Delta z k_{m12}(u_2(z,t)-k_{e12}u_1(z,t))$$

$$-(1-\epsilon)A_c\Delta z r_2 u_2(z,t)^{n_2} \tag{A2.1}$$

An explanation of the terms in eq. (A2.1) follows.

- $(1-\epsilon)A_c\Delta z\dfrac{\partial u_2(z,t)}{\partial t}$: Change in the primary protein concentration with t. The units of the term are:

$$(\frac{cm_c^3}{cm_l^3})(cm_l^2)(cm_l)\left(\frac{primary\ protein\ concentration}{cm_c^3-sec}\right)$$
$$=\frac{primary\ protein\ concentration}{sec}$$

- $-(1-\epsilon)A_c\Delta z k_{m12}(u_2(z,t)-k_{e12}u_1(z,t))$: Rate of transfer of virus to host cells. The units of the term are:

$$(\frac{cm_c^3}{cm_l^3})(cm_l^2)(cm_l)\frac{1}{sec}\left(\frac{primary\ protein\ concentration}{cm_c^3}\right.$$
$$-\frac{\dfrac{primary\ protein\ concentration}{cm_c^3}}{\dfrac{virus\ population}{cm_a^3}}\left.\frac{virus\ population}{cm_a^3}\right)$$
$$=\frac{primary\ protein\ concentration}{sec}$$

The mass transfer term, $-k_{m12}(u_2(z,t)-k_{e12}u_1(z,t))$, involves the difference of the primary protein concentration (in the cells) and the virus population (in the air passage).
- $-(1-\epsilon)A_c\Delta z r_2 u_2(z,t)^{n_2}$: Volumetric rate of production of the secondary protein in the host cells from the primary

protein. The units of the term are:

$$(\frac{cm_c^3}{cm_l^3})(cm_l^2)(cm_l)(\frac{(cm_c^3)^{(n_2-1)}}{(primary\ protein\ concentration)^{(n_2-1)} - sec} \cdot \left(\frac{primary\ protein\ concentration}{cm_c^3}\right)^{n_2})$$

$$= (cm_c^3)(\frac{(cm_c^3)^{(n_2-1)}}{(primary\ protein\ concentration)^{(n_2-1)} - sec} \cdot \left(\frac{primary\ protein\ concentration}{cm_c^3}\right)^{n_2})$$

$$= \frac{primary\ protein\ concentration}{sec}$$

The units of r_2 are dependent on the value of n_2. For example,

- For $n_2 = 1$ (a first order production rate for the secondary protein), the units of r_2 are $\frac{1}{sec}$.
- For $n_2 = 2$ (a second order production rate for the secondary protein), the units of r_2 are

$$\frac{cm_c^3}{(primary\ protein\ concentration) - sec}.$$

Variation in r_2 and n_2 is left as an exercise.

Minor rearrangement of eq. (A2.1) gives

$$\frac{\partial u_2(z,t)}{\partial t} =$$

$$-k_{m12}(u_2(z,t) - k_{e12}u_1(z,t))$$

$$-r_2 u_2(z,t)^{n_2} \tag{A2.2}$$

Eq. (A2.2) is eq. (1.1-2).

The derivation of the $u_3(z,t)$ PDE, eq. (1.1-3), is based on a secondary protein balance for an incremental volume

$(1 - \epsilon)A_c\Delta z.$

$$(1 - \epsilon)A_c\Delta z\frac{\partial u_3(z,t)}{\partial t} =$$

$$-(1 - \epsilon)A_c\Delta z k_{m12}(u_3(z,t) - \frac{1}{k_{e34}}u_4(z,t))$$

$$+(1 - \epsilon)A_c\Delta z r_2 u_2(z,t)^{n_2} \qquad (A3.1)$$

An explanation of the terms in eq. (A3.1) follows.

- $(1 - \epsilon)A_c\Delta z\dfrac{\partial u_3(z,t)}{\partial t}$: Change in the secondary protein concentration with t. The units of the terms, with $k_{m34} = \dfrac{1}{sec}$,

$$k_{e34} = \frac{\dfrac{virion\ population}{cm_a^3}}{\dfrac{secondary\ protein\ concentration}{cm_c^3}}, \text{ are:}$$

$$(\frac{cm_c^3}{cm_l^3})(cm_l^2)(cm_l)\left(\frac{secondary\ protein\ concentration}{cm_c^3 - sec}\right)$$

$$= \frac{secondary\ protein\ concentration}{sec}$$

- $-(1 - \epsilon)A_c\Delta z k_{m34}(u_3(z,t) - \dfrac{1}{k_{e34}}u_4(z,t))$: Rate of transfer of host cells to virions. The units of the term are:

$$(\frac{cm_c^3}{cm_l^3})(cm_l^2)(cm_l)\frac{1}{sec}\left(\frac{secondary\ protein\ concentration}{cm_c^3}\right.$$

$$\left. - \frac{\dfrac{secondary\ protein\ concentration}{cm_c^3}}{\dfrac{virion\ population}{cm_a^3}}\frac{viron\ population}{cm_a^3}\right)$$

$$= \frac{scondary\ protein\ concentration}{sec}$$

The mass transfer term, $-k_{m34}(u_3(z,t) - \dfrac{1}{k_{e34}}u_4(z,t))$, is based on the difference of the secondary protein concentration (in the cells) and the virion population (in the air passage).

- $(1-\epsilon)A_c\Delta z r_2 u_2(z,t)^{n_2}$: Volumetric rate of production of the secondary protein in the host cells from the primary protein. The units of this term are the same as for this term in eq. (A2.1)[2].

Minor rearrangement of eq. (A3.1) gives

$$\frac{\partial u_3(z,t)}{\partial t} =$$

$$-k_{m34}(u_4(z,t) - \frac{1}{k_{e12}}u_4(z,t))$$

$$+r_2 u_2(z,t)^{n_2} \tag{A3.2}$$

Eq. (A3.2) is eq. (1.1-3).

The derivation of the $u_4(z,t)$ PDE, eq. (1.1-4), is based on a virion population balance for an incremental volume $\epsilon A_c \Delta z$.

$$\epsilon A_c \Delta z \frac{\partial u_4(z,t)}{\partial t} =$$

$$v_1(z,t)\epsilon A_c u_4(z,t)|_{z-\Delta z} - v_1(z,t)\epsilon A_c u_4(z,t)|_z$$

$$+\epsilon A_c \Delta z k_{34}(k_{e34}u_3(z,t) - u_4(z,t)) \tag{A4.1}$$

An explanation of the terms in eq. (A4.1) follows.

---

[2]A unit stoichiometric coefficient between the primary and secondary proteins is assumed. Another value for the stoichiometric coefficient can be used at this point to relate the term $(1-\epsilon)A_c\Delta z r_2 u_2(z,t)^{n_2}$ in eqs. (A2.1) and (A3.1).

- $\epsilon A_c \Delta z \dfrac{\partial u_4(z,t)}{\partial t}$: Change in the virion population with t. The units of the term are:

$$(\frac{cm_a^3}{cm_l^3})(cm_l^2)(cm_l)\left(\frac{virion\ population}{cm_a^3 - sec}\right) = \frac{virion\ population}{sec}$$

In summary, the net units are $\dfrac{virion\ population}{sec}$.

- $v_1(z,t)\epsilon A_c u_4(z,t)|_{z-\Delta z}$: Virions entering the incremental volume at $z - \Delta z$. The units of the term are:

$$(\frac{cm_l}{sec})(\frac{cm_a^3}{cm_l^3})(cm_l^2)\left(\frac{virion\ population}{cm_a^3}\right) = \frac{virion\ population}{sec}$$

The convective term at z has the same units as $\dfrac{\partial u_4}{\partial t}$ above.

- $\epsilon A_c \Delta z k_{34}(k_{e34}u_3(z,t) - u_4(z,t))$: Rate of transfer of host cells to virions. The units of the term are:

$$(\frac{cm_a^3}{cm_l^3})(cm_l^2)(cm_l^2)(cm_l)\frac{1}{sec}$$

$$\left(\frac{\dfrac{virion\ population}{cm_a^3}}{\dfrac{secondary\ protein\ concentration}{cm_c^3}}\right.$$

$$\left.\frac{secondary\ protein\ concentration}{cm_c^3} - \frac{virion\ population}{cm_a^3}\right)$$

$$= \frac{virion\ population}{sec}$$

The mass transfer term, $k_{m34}(k_{e34}u_3(z,t) - u_4(z,t))$, is based on the difference of the secondary protein concentration (in the cells) and the virion population (in the air passage).

Minor rearrangement of eq. (A4.1) gives

$$\frac{\partial u_4(z,t)}{\partial t} =$$

$$-\left(\frac{v_1(z,t)u_4(z,t)|_z - v_1(z,t)u_4(z,t)|_{z-\Delta z}}{\Delta z} \\ +k_{34}(k_{e34}u_3(z,t) - u_4(z,t)) \right) \tag{A4.2}$$

In the limit $\Delta z \to 0$, eq. (A4.2) is

$$\frac{\partial u_4(z,t)}{\partial t} = -\left(\frac{\partial v_1(z,t)u_4(z,t)}{\partial z} \right) + k_{34}(k_{e34}u_3(z,t) - u_4(z,t)) \tag{A4.3}$$

For $v_1(z,t) = v_1(t)$, eq. (A4.3) is eq. (1.1-4).

Chapter 2

Lung/Respiratory System Model Implementation

(2) Introduction

The 4×4 PDE model formulated in Chapter 1, eqs. (1.1), (1.2), (1.3), is implemented in this chapter.

(2.1) PDE model implementation

The numerical integration (solution) of the four PDE model, eqs. (1.1), (1.2), (1.3), is implemented in the following R routines, starting with a main program.

(2.1.1) Main program

A main program for eqs. (1.1), (1.2), (1.3) follows.

```
#
# Four PDE model
#
# Delete previous workspaces
  rm(list=ls(all=TRUE))
#
# Access ODE integrator
  library("deSolve");
#
# Access functions for numerical solution
```

```
setwd("f:/chap2");
source("pde1a.R");
#
# Parameters
  u1e=1;
  r2=1;
  n2=1;
  ke12=1;
  ke34=1;
  km12=0.1;
  km34=0.1;
  u10=0;
  u20=0;
  u30=0;
  u40=0;
  ncase=1;
#
# Spatial grid (in z)
  nz=41;zl=0;zu=20;dz=(zu-zl)/(nz-1)
  z=seq(from=zl,to=zu,by=dz);
#
# Independent variable for ODE integration
  t0=0;tf=1;nout=21;
  tout=seq(from=t0,to=tf,by=(tf-t0)/(nout-1));
#
# Initial condition (t=0)
  u0=rep(0,4*nz);
  for(i in 1:nz){
    u0[i]      =u10;
    u0[i+nz]   =u20;
    u0[i+2*nz]=u30;
    u0[i+3*nz]=u40;
  }
  ncall=0;
```

```
#
# ODE integration
  out=lsodes(y=u0,times=tout,func=pde1a,
      sparsetype ="sparseint",rtol=1e-6,
      atol=1e-6,maxord=5);
  nrow(out)
  ncol(out)
#
# Arrays for plotting numerical solution
  u1=matrix(0,nrow=nz,ncol=nout);
  u2=matrix(0,nrow=nz,ncol=nout);
  u3=matrix(0,nrow=nz,ncol=nout);
  u4=matrix(0,nrow=nz,ncol=nout);
  for(it in 1:nout){
    for(i in 1:nz){
      u1[i,it]=out[it,i+1];
      u2[i,it]=out[it,i+1+nz];
      u3[i,it]=out[it,i+1+2*nz];
      u4[i,it]=out[it,i+1+3*nz];
    }
  }
#
# Display numerical solution
  iv=seq(from=1,to=nout,by=10);
  for(it in iv){
    if(ncase==1)
      {v1=40*sin(  pi*(tout[it]-t0)/(tf-t0));}
    if(ncase==2)
      {v1=40*sin(2*pi*(tout[it]-t0)/(tf-t0));}
    if(v1>=0){
      u1[1,it]=u1e;
      u4[1,it]=0;}
    cat(sprintf(
      "\n t = %6.2f v1 = %6.2f\n",tout[it],v1));
```

```
    iv=seq(from=1,to=nz,by=10);
    for(i in iv){
      cat(sprintf("%6.1f%6.1f%12.3e\n",
          tout[it],z[i],u1[i,it]));
    }
    cat(sprintf("\n    t     z     u2(z,t)\n"));
    iv=seq(from=1,to=nz,by=10);
    for(i in iv){
      cat(sprintf("%6.1f%6.1f%12.3e\n",
          tout[it],z[i],u2[i,it]));
    }
    cat(sprintf("\n    t     z     u3(z,t)\n"));
    iv=seq(from=1,to=nz,by=10);
    for(i in iv){
      cat(sprintf("%6.1f%6.1f%12.3e\n",
          tout[it],z[i],u3[i,it]));
    }
    cat(sprintf("\n    t     z     u4(z,t)\n"));
    iv=seq(from=1,to=nz,by=10);
    for(i in iv){
      cat(sprintf("%6.1f%6.1f%12.3e\n",
          tout[it],z[i],u4[i,it]));
    }
  }
#
# Calls to ODE routine
  cat(sprintf("\n\n ncall = %5d\n\n",ncall));
#
# Plot PDE solutions
#
# u1(z,t)
# 2D
  par(mfrow=c(1,1));
  matplot(x=z[2:nz],y=u1[2:nz,],type="l",xlab="z",
```

```
   ylab="u1(z,t)",xlim=c(zl,zu),lty=1,main="",
   lwd=2,col="black");
#
# 3D
  persp(z,tout,u1,theta=45,phi=30,
        xlim=c(zl,zu),ylim=c(t0,tf),xlab="z",
        ylab="t",zlab="u1(z,t)");
#
# u2(z,t)
# 2D
  par(mfrow=c(1,1));
  matplot(x=z[2:nz],y=u2[2:nz,],type="l",xlab="z",
    ylab="u2(z,t)",xlim=c(zl,zu),lty=1,main="",
    lwd=2,col="black");
#
# 3D
  persp(z,tout,u2,theta=60,phi=30,
        xlim=c(zl,zu),ylim=c(t0,tf),xlab="z",
        ylab="t",zlab="u2(z,t)");
#
# u3(z,t)
# 2D
  par(mfrow=c(1,1));
  matplot(x=z,y=u3,type="l",xlab="z",
    ylab="u3(z,t)",xlim=c(zl,zu),lty=1,
    main="",lwd=2,col="black");
#
# 3D
  persp(z,tout,u3,theta=60,phi=30,
        xlim=c(zl,zu),ylim=c(t0,tf),xlab="z",
        ylab="t",zlab="u3(z,t)");
#
# u4(z,t)
# 2D
```

```
par(mfrow=c(1,1));
matplot(x=z,y=u4,type="l",xlab="z",
   ylab="u4(z,t)",xlim=c(zl,zu),lty=1,
   main="",lwd=2,col="black");
```
```
#
# 3D
persp(z,tout,u4,theta=60,phi=30,
      xlim=c(zl,zu),ylim=c(t0,tf),xlab="z",
      ylab="t",zlab="u4(z,t)");
```

Listing 2.1: Main program for eqs. (1.1), (1.2), (1.3)

We can note the following details about Listing 2.1.

- Previous workspaces are deleted.

```
#
# Four PDE model
#
# Delete previous workspaces
  rm(list=ls(all=TRUE))
```

- The R ODE integrator library deSolve is accessed [2]. Then the directory with the files for the solution of eqs. (1.1) is designated. Note that setwd (set working directory) uses / rather than the usual \.

```
#
# Access ODE integrator
  library("deSolve");
#
# Access functions for numerical solution
  setwd("f:/chap2");
  source("pde1a.R");
```

pde1a is the ODE/MOL routine for eqs. (1.1), (1.2), (1.3), discussed subsequently.

- The model parameters are specified numerically.

```
#
# Parameters
  u1e=1;
  r2=1;
  n2=1;
  ke12=1;
  ke34=1;
  km12=0.1;
  km34=0.1;
  u10=0;
  u20=0;
  u30=0;
  u40=0;
  ncase=1;
```

The parameters are named in analogy with eqs. (1.1), (1.2), (1.3). For example, $km12 = k_{m12}$ in eqs. (1.1-1,2), $km34 = k_{m34}$ in eqs. (1.1-3,4), $r2,n2 = r_2, n_2$ in eqs. (1.1-2,3), The initial conditions (ICs) are $u10,u20,u30,u40 = u_{10}(z)$, $u_{20}(z)$, $u_{30}(z)$, $u_{40}(z)$ in eqs. (1.2). The boundary condition (BC) function $u1e = u_1(z = 0, t) = u_{1b}(t)$ is in eq. (1.3-1).

ncase selects a case for $v_1(t)$, (1) $v_1(t) > 0$ (ncase=1), or (2) switching of the air flow direction, $v_1(t) > 0, < 0$ (ncase=2), as explained in the discussion of pde1a.

- A spatial grid for eqs. (1.1) is defined with 41 points so that z = 0,0.5,...,20. The air passage length is $z_u = 20$ cm.

```
#
# Spatial grid (in z)
  nz=41;zl=0;zu=20;dz=(zu-zl)/(nz-1)
  z=seq(from=zl,to=zu,by=dz);
```

- An interval in t is defined for 21 output points, so that tout=0,1/20,...,1 (sec).

```
#
# Independent variable for ODE integration
  t0=0;tf=1;nout=21;
  tout=seq(from=t0,to=tf,by=(tf-t0)/(nout-1));
```

- ICs (1.2) are implemented. $u_1(z, t = 0)$ is placed in a vector u0[i] of length nz, then $u_2(z, t = 0)$ is added to u0, etc., for $u_3(z, t = 0)$, $u_4(z, t = 0)$.

```
#
# Initial condition (t=0)
  u0=rep(0,4*nz);
  for(i in 1:nz){
     u0[i]      =u10;
     u0[i+nz]   =u20;
     u0[i+2*nz]=u30;
     u0[i+3*nz]=u40;
  }
  ncall=0;
```

Also, the counter for the calls to pde1a is initialized.

- The system of $(4)41 = 164$ ODEs is integrated by the library integrator lsodes (available in deSolve, [2]). As expected, the inputs to lsodes are the ODE function, pde1a, the IC vector u0, and the vector of output values of t, tout. The length of u0 (164) informs lsodes how many ODEs are to be integrated. func,y,times are reserved names.

```
#
# ODE integration
  out=lsodes(y=u0,times=tout,func=pde1a,
       sparsetype ="sparseint",rtol=1e-6,
```

```
     atol=1e-6,maxord=5);
  nrow(out)
  ncol(out)
```

nrow,ncol confirm the dimensions of out.
- $u_1(z,t)$, $u_2(z,t)$, $u_3(z,t)$, $u_4(z,t)$ are placed in matrices for subsequent plotting.

```
#
# Arrays for plotting numerical solution
  u1=matrix(0,nrow=nz,ncol=nout);
  u2=matrix(0,nrow=nz,ncol=nout);
  u3=matrix(0,nrow=nz,ncol=nout);
  u4=matrix(0,nrow=nz,ncol=nout);
  for(it in 1:nout){
    for(i in 1:nz){
      u1[i,it]=out[it,i+1];
      u2[i,it]=out[it,i+1+nz];
      u3[i,it]=out[it,i+1+2*nz];
      u4[i,it]=out[it,i+1+3*nz];
    }
  }
```

The offset +1 is required since the first element of the solution vectors in out is the value of t and the 2 to 165 elements are the 4(41) values of $u_1(z,t)$, $u_2(z,t)$, $u_3(z,t)$, $u_4(z,t)$. These dimensions from the preceding calls to nrow,ncol are confirmed in the subsequent output.
- The values of $u_1(z,t)$ are displayed as a function of z and t with two fors. Within the t for with index it, ncase selects the velocity $v_1(t)$ as explained subsequently. For $v_1(t) > 0$, the boundary values $u_1(z = 0, t) =$ u1[1,it], $u_4(z = 0, t) =$ u4[1,it] are set according to BCs (1.3-1,2).

```
#
# Display numerical solution
  iv=seq(from=1,to=nout,by=10);
  for(it in iv){
    if(ncase==1)
      {v1=40*sin(  pi*(tout[it]-t0)/(tf-t0));}
    if(ncase==2)
      {v1=40*sin(2*pi*(tout[it]-t0)/(tf-t0));}
    if(v1>=0){
      u1[1,it]=u1e;
      u4[1,it]=0;}
    cat(sprintf(
      "\n t = %6.2f v1 = %6.2f\n",tout[it],v1));
    cat(sprintf("\n    t    z      u1(z,t)\n"));
    iv=seq(from=1,to=nz,by=10);
    for(i in iv){
      cat(sprintf("%6.1f%6.1f%12.3e\n",
          tout[it],z[i],u1[i,it]));
    }
```

Every tenth value of $u_1(z,t)$ is displayed in z, t with by=10.

- $u_2(z,t)$, $u_3(z,t)$, $u_4(z,t)$ are displayed in the same way as $u_1(z,t)$.

```
    cat(sprintf("\n    t    z      u2(z,t)\n"));
    iv=seq(from=1,to=nz,by=10);
    for(i in iv){
      cat(sprintf("%6.1f%6.1f%12.3e\n",
          tout[it],z[i],u2[i,it]));
    }
    cat(sprintf("\n    t    z      u3(z,t)\n"));
    iv=seq(from=1,to=nz,by=10);
    for(i in iv){
      cat(sprintf("%6.1f%6.1f%12.3e\n",
```

```
         tout[it],z[i],u3[i,it]));
    }
    cat(sprintf("\n     t      z      u4(z,t)\n"));
    iv=seq(from=1,to=nz,by=10);
    for(i in iv){
      cat(sprintf("%6.1f%6.1f%12.3e\n",
         tout[it],z[i],u4[i,it]));
    }
  }
```

The final } ends the **for** in t (with index **it**).

- The total number of calls to **pde1a** is displayed.

```
#
# Calls to ODE routine
    cat(sprintf("\n\n ncall = %5d\n\n",ncall));
```

- The solutions $u_1(z,t)$, $u_2(z,t)$, $u_3(z,t)$, $u_4(z,t)$ are plotted in 2D with the utility **matplot** and in 3D with the utility **persp**. For $u_1(z,t)$, $u_2(z,t)$ the solutions at $z = z_l = 0$ are not included, **x=z[2:nz]**, to avoid the distortion of the discontinuous change from ICs (1.2-1,2) to BC (1.3-1) as explained subsequently. Including $u_1(z = z_l = 0, t)$, $u_2(z = z_l = 0, t)$ is left as an exercise.

```
#
# Plot PDE solutions
#
# u1(z,t)
# 2D
    par(mfrow=c(1,1));
    matplot(x=z[2:nz],y=u1[2:nz,],type="l",xlab="z",
       ylab="u1(z,t)",xlim=c(zl,zu),lty=1,main="",
       lwd=2,col="black");
#
# 3D
```

```
      persp(z,tout,u1,theta=45,phi=30,
            xlim=c(zl,zu),ylim=c(t0,tf),xlab="z",
            ylab="t",zlab="u1(z,t)");
#
# u2(z,t)
# 2D
    par(mfrow=c(1,1));
    matplot(x=z[2:nz],y=u2[2:nz,],type="l",xlab="z",
      ylab="u2(z,t)",xlim=c(zl,zu),lty=1,main="",
      lwd=2,col="black");
#
# 3D
    persp(z,tout,u2,theta=60,phi=30,
            xlim=c(zl,zu),ylim=c(t0,tf),xlab="z",
            ylab="t",zlab="u2(z,t)");
#
# u3(z,t)
# 2D
    par(mfrow=c(1,1));
    matplot(x=z,y=u3,type="l",xlab="z",
      ylab="u3(z,t)",xlim=c(zl,zu),lty=1,
      main="",lwd=2,col="black");
#
# 3D
    persp(z,tout,u3,theta=60,phi=30,
            xlim=c(zl,zu),ylim=c(t0,tf),xlab="z",
            ylab="t",zlab="u3(z,t)");
#
# u4(z,t)
# 2D
    par(mfrow=c(1,1));
    matplot(x=z,y=u4,type="l",xlab="z",
      ylab="u4(z,t)",xlim=c(zl,zu),lty=1,
      main="",lwd=2,col="black");
```

```
#
#  3D
   persp(z,tout,u4,theta=60,phi=30,
           xlim=c(zl,zu),ylim=c(t0,tf),xlab="z",
           ylab="t",zlab="u4(z,t)");
```

This completes the discussion of the main program in Listing 2.1. The ODE/PDE routine called by `lsodes` in the main program is considered next.

(2.1.2) ODE/MOL routine

The ODE/MOL routine for eqs. (1.1), (1.2), (1.3) follows.

```
pde1a=function(t,u,parm){
#
# Function pde1a computes the t derivatives
# of u1(z,t),u2(z,t),u3(z,t),u4(z,t)
#
# One vector to four vectors
  u1=rep(0,nz);
  u2=rep(0,nz);
  u3=rep(0,nz);
  u4=rep(0,nz);
  for(i in 1:nz){
    u1[i]=u[i];
    u2[i]=u[i+nz];
    u3[i]=u[i+2*nz];
    u4[i]=u[i+3*nz];
  }
#
# PDE t vectors
  u1t=rep(0,nz);
  u2t=rep(0,nz);
  u3t=rep(0,nz);
```

```
    u4t=rep(0,nz);
#
# v1(t) for ncase=1,2
  if(ncase==1){
    v1=40*sin(  pi*(t-t0)/(tf-t0));}
  if(ncase==2){
    v1=40*sin(2*pi*(t-t0)/(tf-t0));}
#
# v1(t)>=0
  if(v1>=0){
#
# BCs
    u1[1]=u1e;
    u4[1]=0;
    u1t[1]=0;
    u4t[1]=0;
#
# PDEs for u1(z,t), u4(z,t)
    for(i in 2:nz){
      u1t[i]=-v1*(u1[i]-u1[i-1])/dz+
             km12*((1/ke12)*u2[i]-u1[i]);
      u4t[i]=-v1*(u4[i]-u4[i-1])/dz+
             km34*(ke34*u3[i]-u4[i]);
    }
  }
#
# v1(t)<0
  if(v1<0){
#
# BCs
    u1t[nz]=km12*((1/ke12)*u2[nz]-u1[nz]);
    u4t[nz]=km34*(ke34*u3[nz]-u4[nz]);
#
# PDEs for u1(z,t), u4(z,t)
```

```r
  for(i in 1:(nz-1)){
    u1t[i]=-v1*(u1[i+1]-u1[i])/dz+
           km12*((1/ke12)*u2[i]-u1[i]);
    u4t[i]=-v1*(u4[i+1]-u4[i])/dz+
           km34*(ke34*u3[i]-u4[i]);
    }
  }
#
# PDEs for u2(z,t), u3(z,t)
  for(i in 1:nz){
    u2t[i]=-km12*(u2[i]-ke12*u1[i])-
           r2*u2[i]^n2;
    u3t[i]=-km34*(u3[i]-(1/ke34)*u4[i])+
           r2*u2[i]^n2;
    }
#
# Four vectors to one vector
  ut=rep(0,4*nz);
  for(i in 1:nz){
    ut[i]      =u1t[i];
    ut[i+nz]   =u2t[i];
    ut[i+2*nz]=u3t[i];
    ut[i+3*nz]=u4t[i];
    }
#
# Increment calls to pde1a
  ncall <<- ncall+1;
#
# Return derivative vector
  return(list(c(ut)));
  }
```

Listing 2.2: ODE/MOL routine for eqs. (1.1), (1.2), (1.3)

We can note the following details about pde1a.

- The function is defined.

```
pde1a=function(t,u,parm){
#
# Function pde1a computes the t derivatives
# of u1(z,t),u2(z,t),u3(z,t),u4(z,t)
```

  t is the current value of t in eqs. (1.1). u is the 164-vector of ODE/PDE dependent variables. parm is an argument to pass parameters to pde1a (unused, but required in the argument list). The arguments must be listed in the order stated to properly interface with lsodes called in the main program of Listing 2.1. The derivative vector of the LHS of eqs. (1.1) is calculated and returned to lsodes as explained subsequently.

- Vector u is placed in four vectors to facilitate the programming of eqs. (1.1), (1.3).

```
#
# One vector to four vectors
  u1=rep(0,nz);
  u2=rep(0,nz);
  u3=rep(0,nz);
  u4=rep(0,nz);
  for(i in 1:nz){
    u1[i]=u[i];
    u2[i]=u[i+nz];
    u3[i]=u[i+2*nz];
    u4[i]=u[i+3*nz];
  }
```

- Vectors are defined for $\dfrac{\partial u_1(z,t)}{\partial t}$, $\dfrac{\partial u_2(z,t)}{\partial t}$, $\dfrac{\partial u_3(z,t)}{\partial t}$, $\dfrac{\partial u_4(z,t)}{\partial t}$.

```
#
# PDE t vectors
  u1t=rep(0,nz);
  u2t=rep(0,nz);
  u3t=rep(0,nz);
  u4t=rep(0,nz);
```

- The velocity $v_1(t)$ in eqs. (1.1-1,4) is a sin function which gives a smooth increase, then decrease, in t. For ncase=2, the air flow can reverse for inhalation followed by exhalation.

```
#
# Inhalation, exhalation
  if(ncase==1){
    v1=40*sin(  pi*(t-t0)/(tf-t0));}
  if(ncase==2){
    v1=40*sin(2*pi*(t-t0)/(tf-t0));}
```

For ncase=1, $v_1(t) > 0$ over a half sin cycle for $t_0 = 0 \le t \le t_f = 1$ ($t_0 = 0, t_f = 1$ are set numerically in the main program of Listing 2.1). For ncase=2, $v_1(t) > 0$ over a half sin cycle for $t_0 = 0 \le t \le t_f/2 = 0.5$, then $v_1(t) < 0$ over a half sin cycle for $t_f/2 = 0.5 < t \le t_f = 1$.

As a variation on this calculation for ncase=2, the amplitude of $v_1(t)$ could be different for $0 \le t \le 0.5$ and $0.5 < t \le 1$. For example, if the air passage effective cross sectional area, A_c, is different for inhalation and exhalation, the amplitude $v_1 = 40$ could be adjusted so that the product $A_c v_1$, that is, the volumetric flow rate in the air passage, remains the same for inhalation and exhalation. This variation of $v_1(t)$ is left as an exercise.

- For $v_1(t) >= 0$ (inhalation), the coding is in a if.

```
#
# v1(t)>=0
  if(v1>=0){
```

- BCs (1.3-1,2) are defined algebraically. The derivatives in t are set to zero to prevent any departure of the BCs from the prescribed values.

```
#
# BCs
    u1[1]=u1e;
    u4[1]=0;
    u1t[1]=0;
    u4t[1]=0;
```

- Eqs. (1.1-1,4) are coded in the MOL format.

```
#
# PDEs for u1(z,t), u4(z,t)
    for(i in 2:nz){
      u1t[i]=-v1*(u1[i]-u1[i-1])/dz+
             km12*((1/ke12)*u2[i]-u1[i]);
      u4t[i]=-v1*(u4[i]-u4[i-1])/dz+
             km34*(ke34*u3[i]-u4[i]);
    }
  }
```

The for in z does not include $z = z_l = 0$ since this point is programmed separately as BCs. The final } concludes the if for $v_1(t) >= 0$.

- For $v_1(t) < 0$ (exhalation), the coding is in a if.

```
#
# v1(t)<0
  if(v1<0){
```

- BCs (1.3-3,4) are defined as ODEs in t. These BCs are eqs. (1.1-1,4) with no convection ($v_1(t) = 0$ at $z = z_u = 20$ cm).

```
#
# BCs
    u1t[nz]=km12*((1/ke12)*u2[nz]-u1[nz]);
    u4t[nz]=km34*(ke34*u3[nz]-u4[nz]);
```

- Eqs. (1.1-1,4) are coded in the MOL format.

```
#
# PDEs for u1(z,t), u4(z,t)
    for(i in 1:(nz-1)){
      u1t[i]=-v1*(u1[i+1]-u1[i])/dz+
             km12*((1/ke12)*u2[i]-u1[i]);
      u4t[i]=-v1*(u4[i+1]-u4[i])/dz+
             km34*(ke34*u3[i]-u4[i]);
    }
  }
```

The `for` in z does not include $z = z_u = 20$ since this point is programmed separately as BCs. The final } concludes the `if` for $v_1(t) <$.

The partial derivatives in z in eqs. (1.1-1,4), $\dfrac{\partial u_1}{\partial z}$, $\dfrac{\partial u_4}{\partial z}$, are approximated by two-point upwind finite differences (FDs).

For $v_1(t) >= 0$,

$$\frac{\partial u_1}{\partial z} \approx \frac{u_1(z,t) - u_1(z - \Delta z, t)}{\Delta z}$$

$$\frac{\partial u_4}{\partial z} \approx \frac{u_4(z,t) - u_4(z - \Delta z, t)}{\Delta z}$$

For $v_1(t) < 0$,

$$\frac{\partial u_1}{\partial z} \approx \frac{u_1(z + \Delta z, t) - u_1(z,t)}{\Delta z}$$

$$\frac{\partial u_4}{\partial z} \approx \frac{u_4(z + \Delta z, t) - u_4(z,t)}{\Delta z}$$

These FD approximations are first order correct in Δz, designated as $O(\Delta z)$. While they are generally stable and produce smooth solutions, they also introduce substantial numerical diffusion (dispersion) in z. Here we assume nz=41 is sufficient to keep the numerical diffusion to an acceptable level.

Higher order approximations of the spatial (convective) derivatives are discussed in [1]. These approximations include higher order FDs, which reduce numerical diffusion but introduce numerical oscillation, and flux limiter approximations. The latter give good resolution of steep moving fronts and discontinuities (minimal numerical diffusion) with no numerical oscillation.

Eqs. (1.1-1,4) are termed *first order hyperbolic PDEs*. The numerical solution of hyperbolic PDEs has an extensive literature and will not be considered further in this discussion. For the present model, the smooth (sin) variation in $v_1(t)$ limits numerical diffusion and oscillation. The effect of nz in the preceding R analysis is left as an exercise.

- Eqs. (1.1-2,3) are programmed in the MOL format.

```
#
# PDEs for u2(z,t), u3(z,t)
  for(i in 1:nz){
    u2t[i]=-km12*(u2[i]-ke12*u1[i])-
           r2*u2[i]^n2;
    u3t[i]=-km34*(u3[i]-(1/ke34)*u4[i])+
           r2*u2[i]^n2;
  }
```

Note that eqs. (1.1-2,3) are PDEs even though they do not include spatial derivatives in z. That is, $u_2(z,t), u_3(z,t)$ are functions of z and t and require approximation on a spatial grid in z.

- u1t, u2t, u3t, u4t are placed in a single vector, ut, for return to lsodes to take the next step in t along the solution.

```
#
# Four vectors to one vector
  ut=rep(0,4*nz);
  for(i in 1:nz){
    ut[i]     =u1t[i];
    ut[i+nz]  =u2t[i];
    ut[i+2*nz]=u3t[i];
    ut[i+3*nz]=u4t[i];
  }
```

- The number of calls to pde1a is incremented and returned to the main program of Listing 2.1 with <<-.

```
#
# Increment calls to pde1a
  ncall <<- ncall+1;
```

- The derivative vector ut is returned to lsodes as a list as required by lsodes.

```
#
# Return derivative vector
  return(list(c(ut)));
  }
```

c is the R numerical vector operator.

This completes the discussion of pde1a. Two tests of the coding in Listings 2.1, 2.2 can easily be applied: (1) For $u_{1b}(t) =$ u1e=0 in BC (1.3-1), there is no virus source, and the dependent variables $u_1(z,t), u_2(z,t), u_3(z,t), u_4(z,t)$ remain at zero (homogeneous) ICs (ICs (1.2) with zero functions), and (2) For $r_2 =$ r2=0, $u_3(z,t), u_4(z,t)$ remain at zero ICs (no secondary protein and virions are produced). If in (1) and (2) the indicated PDE dependent variables do not remain at zero ICs, an error in the model and/or coding is indicated. These tests are left as an exercise.

The numerical and graphical output from the R routines of Listings 2.1, 2.2 is considered next.

(2.1.3) Numerical and graphical output

The numerical output for ncase=1 follows.

```
[1] 21

[1] 165
```

```
t =    0.00 v1 =    0.00
```

t	z	u1(z,t)
0.0	0.0	1.000e+00
0.0	5.0	0.000e+00
0.0	10.0	0.000e+00
0.0	15.0	0.000e+00
0.0	20.0	0.000e+00
t	z	u2(z,t)
0.0	0.0	0.000e+00
0.0	5.0	0.000e+00
0.0	10.0	0.000e+00
0.0	15.0	0.000e+00
0.0	20.0	0.000e+00

t	z	u3(z,t)
0.0	0.0	0.000e+00
0.0	5.0	0.000e+00
0.0	10.0	0.000e+00
0.0	15.0	0.000e+00
0.0	20.0	0.000e+00

```
  t      z      u4(z,t)
 0.0    0.0    0.000e+00
 0.0    5.0    0.000e+00
 0.0   10.0    0.000e+00
 0.0   15.0    0.000e+00
 0.0   20.0    0.000e+00
```

t =   0.50 v1 =   40.00

```
  t      z      u1(z,t)
 0.5    0.0    1.000e+00
 0.5    5.0    9.872e-01
 0.5   10.0    8.608e-01
 0.5   15.0    2.008e-01
 0.5   20.0    4.459e-03
```

```
  t      z      u2(z,t)
 0.5    0.0    3.846e-02
 0.5    5.0    1.842e-02
 0.5   10.0    6.776e-03
 0.5   15.0    6.396e-04
 0.5   20.0    7.758e-06
```

```
  t      z      u3(z,t)
 0.5    0.0    1.031e-02
 0.5    5.0    2.107e-03
 0.5   10.0    3.702e-04
 0.5   15.0    1.724e-05
 0.5   20.0    1.244e-07
```

```
  t      z      u4(z,t)
 0.5    0.0    0.000e+00
 0.5    5.0    3.275e-05
 0.5   10.0    1.361e-05
```

```
0.5   15.0    1.047e-06
0.5   20.0    1.030e-08


t =    1.00 v1 =    0.00


  t      z      u1(z,t)
1.0    0.0    1.000e+00
1.0    5.0    9.728e-01
1.0   10.0    9.594e-01
1.0   15.0    9.465e-01
1.0   20.0    8.874e-01


  t      z      u2(z,t)
1.0    0.0    6.062e-02
1.0    5.0    4.845e-02
1.0   10.0    4.100e-02
1.0   15.0    3.328e-02
1.0   20.0    2.319e-02


  t      z      u3(z,t)
1.0    0.0    3.451e-02
1.0    5.0    1.908e-02
1.0   10.0    1.279e-02
1.0   15.0    8.034e-03
1.0   20.0    4.063e-03


  t      z      u4(z,t)
1.0    0.0    0.000e+00
1.0    5.0    4.344e-04
1.0   10.0    3.647e-04
1.0   15.0    2.381e-04
1.0   20.0    1.101e-04


ncall =    568
```

Table 2.1: Numerical output from Listings 2.1, 2.2, ncase=1

We can note the following details about this output.

- 21 t output points as the first dimension of the solution matrix out from lsodes as programmed in the main program of Listing 2.1 (with nout=21).
- The solution matrix out returned by lsodes has 165 elements as a second dimension. The first element is the value of t. Elements 2 to 165 are $u_1(z,t)$, $u_2(z,t)$, $u_3(z,t)$, $u_4(z,t)$ $(4(41) = 164$ points in z).
- The solution is displayed for t=0,1/20,...,1 as programmed in Listing 2.1 (every tenth value of t is displayed as explained previously).
- ICs (1.2) are confirmed $(t = 0)$. BC (1.3-1) is also confirmed reflecting the discontinuous change from the IC as discussed previously.

```
   t        z        u1(z,t)
  0.0      0.0      1.000e+00
```

- The velocity $v_1(t = 0.5) = 40$ confirms the sin variation for ncase=1.
- The increase in the secondary protein produced in the host cells is confirmed, e.g.,

```
   t        z        u3(z,t)
  1.0      0.0      3.451e-02
  1.0      5.0      1.908e-02
  1.0     10.0      1.279e-02
  1.0     15.0      8.034e-03
  1.0     20.0      4.063e-03
```

- The increase in the virion population exiting the host cells is confirmed, e.g.,

```
   t        z        u4(z,t)
  1.0      0.0      0.000e+00
  1.0      5.0      4.344e-04
```

```
1.0   10.0    3.647e-04
1.0   15.0    2.381e-04
1.0   20.0    1.101e-04
```

These values are small, but their increase with larger t is of interest in the subsequent discussion.

- The computational effort as indicated by `ncall = 568` is modest so that `lsodes` computed the solution to eqs. (1.1), (1.2), (1.3) efficiently.

The graphical output is in Figs. 2.1.

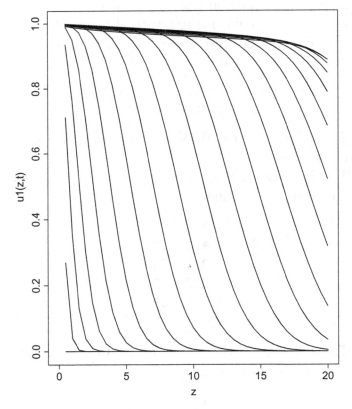

Figure 2.1-1: $u_1(z, t)$ from eq. (1.1-1), 2D from `matplot`, ncase=1

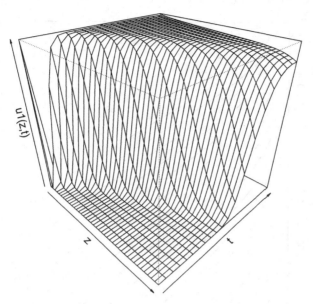

Figure 2.1-2: $u_1(z,t)$ from eq. (1.1-1), 3D from **persp**, **ncase=1**

The solution $u_1(z,t)$ starts from IC (1.2-1), and reflects BC (1.3-1) (at $z = z_l = 0$). The solution $u_1(z = z_l = 0, t)$ is not included as discussed previously.

The solution $u_2(z,t)$ starts from IC (1.2-2), and reflects the response to BC (1.3-1) (at $z = z_l = 0$). The solution $u_2(z = z_l = 0, t)$ is not included as discussed previously.

The solutions in Figs. 2.1-3,4 reflect the invasion of the virus genetic material (VGM) into the host cells.

The solution $u_3(z,t)$ starts from IC (1.2-3), and indicates the production of the secondary protein within the host cell tissue. The increase in $u_3(z,t)$ indicates the infection of the host cells by producton of the secondary protein.

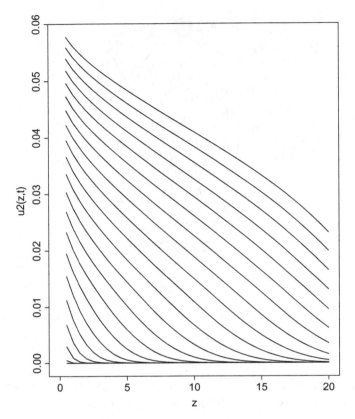

Figure 2.1-3: $u_2(z,t)$ from eq. (1.1-2), 2D from `matplot`, `ncase=1`

The solution $u_4(z,t)$ starts from IC (1.2-4), and indicates the transfer of the secondary protein to the host cell exteriors as virions which can then infect other cells. This transfer therefore represents the spread of the viral infection from the host cells.

Fig 2.1-8 indicates the continuing spread of virions to other host cells.

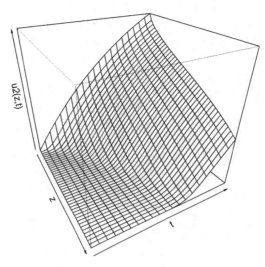

Figure 2.1-4: $u_2(z,t)$ from eq. (1.1-1), 3D from `persp`, `ncase=1`

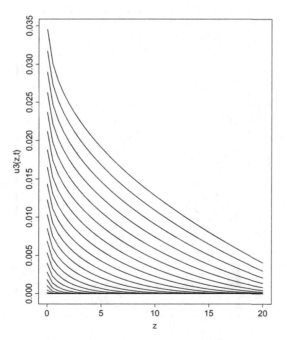

Figure 2.1-5: $u_3(z,t)$ from eq. (1.1-3), 2D from `matplot`, `ncase=1`

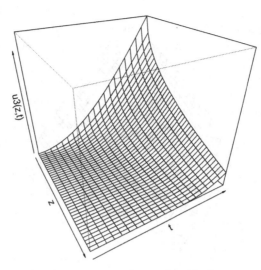

Figure 2.1-6: $u_3(z,t)$ from eq. (1.1-3), 3D from `persp`, ncase=1

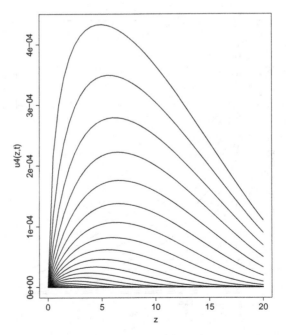

Figure 2.1-7: $u_4(z,t)$ from eq. (1.1-4), 2D from `matplot`, ncase=1

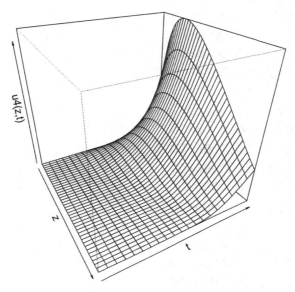

Figure 2.1-8: $u_4(z,t)$ from eq. (1.1-4), 3D from `persp`, `ncase=1`

The numerical output for `ncase=2` follows.

```
[1]  21
```

```
[1]  165
```

```
t =    0.00 v1 =    0.00

    t      z       u1(z,t)
   0.0    0.0    1.000e+00
   0.0    5.0    0.000e+00
   0.0   10.0    0.000e+00
   0.0   15.0    0.000e+00
   0.0   20.0    0.000e+00

    t      z       u2(z,t)
   0.0    0.0    0.000e+00
```

```
0.0    5.0    0.000e+00
0.0   10.0    0.000e+00
0.0   15.0    0.000e+00
0.0   20.0    0.000e+00


 t      z      u3(z,t)
0.0    0.0    0.000e+00
0.0    5.0    0.000e+00
0.0   10.0    0.000e+00
0.0   15.0    0.000e+00
0.0   20.0    0.000e+00


 t      z      u4(z,t)
0.0    0.0    0.000e+00
0.0    5.0    0.000e+00
0.0   10.0    0.000e+00
0.0   15.0    0.000e+00
0.0   20.0    0.000e+00


t =    0.50 v1 =    0.00


 t      z      u1(z,t)
0.5    0.0    1.000e+00
0.5    5.0    9.790e-01
0.5   10.0    8.556e-01
0.5   15.0    2.001e-01
0.5   20.0    4.446e-03


 t      z      u2(z,t)
0.5    0.0    3.846e-02
0.5    5.0    2.407e-02
0.5   10.0    1.275e-02
0.5   15.0    1.801e-03
0.5   20.0    2.908e-05
```

```
  t     z      u3(z,t)
 0.5   0.0   1.031e-02
 0.5   5.0   3.655e-03
 0.5  10.0   1.184e-03
 0.5  15.0   1.055e-04
 0.5  20.0   1.250e-06


  t     z      u4(z,t)
 0.5   0.0   0.000e+00
 0.5   5.0   5.029e-05
 0.5  10.0   1.627e-05
 0.5  15.0   1.162e-06
 0.5  20.0   1.112e-08


t =    1.00 v1 =  -0.00


  t     z      u1(z,t)
 1.0   0.0   4.864e-01
 1.0   5.0   8.468e-02
 1.0  10.0   6.373e-03
 1.0  15.0   4.262e-03
 1.0  20.0   4.235e-03


  t     z      u2(z,t)
 1.0   0.0   4.991e-02
 1.0   5.0   3.417e-02
 1.0  10.0   1.704e-02
 1.0  15.0   2.524e-03
 1.0  20.0   1.833e-04


  t     z      u3(z,t)
 1.0   0.0   3.175e-02
 1.0   5.0   2.036e-02
```

```
1.0   10.0    1.054e-02
1.0   15.0    1.529e-03
1.0   20.0    5.716e-05


 t      z       u4(z,t)
1.0    0.0    6.207e-04
1.0    5.0    3.478e-04
1.0   10.0    1.346e-04
1.0   15.0    1.485e-05
1.0   20.0    1.146e-06


ncall =    616
```

Table 2.2: Numerical output from Listings 2.1, 2.2, `ncase=2`

We can note the following details about this output (with some repetition of the discussion of Table 2.1 so that the following discussion is self contained).

- 21 t output points as the first dimension of the solution matrix out from lsodes as programmed in the main program of Listing 2.1 (with nout=21).
- The solution matrix out returned by lsodes has 165 elements as a second dimension. The first element is the value of t. Elements 2 to 165 are $u_1(z,t)$, $u_2(z,t)$, $u_3(z,t)$, $u_4(z,t)$ $(4(41) = 164$ points in z).
- The solution is displayed for t=0,1/20,...,1 as programmed in Listing 2.1 (every tenth value of t is displayed as explained previously).
- ICs (1.2) are confirmed $(t = 0)$. BC (1.3-1) is also confirmed reflecting the discontinuous change from the IC as discussed previously.

```
 t      z       u1(z,t)
0.0    0.0    1.000e+00
```

- The velocity $v_1(t = 0.5) = 0$ confirms the sin variation for ncase=2.
- The virus population in the air passage is lower for ncase=2 than for ncase=1 as expected (from the exhalation for ncase=2).

ncase=1, Table 2.1

t	z	u1(z,t)
1.0	0.0	1.000e+00
1.0	5.0	9.728e-01
1.0	10.0	9.594e-01
1.0	15.0	9.465e-01
1.0	20.0	8.874e-01

ncase=2, Table 2.2

t	z	u1(z,t)
1.0	0.0	4.864e-01
1.0	5.0	8.468e-02
1.0	10.0	6.373e-03
1.0	15.0	4.262e-03
1.0	20.0	4.235e-03

This reduction for ncase=2 is also confirmed by comparing Figs. 2.1-1,2 with Figs. 2.2-1,2 (that follow).

- The primary protein concentration is also lower for ncase=2 than for ncase=1 as expected (from the exhalation for ncase=2).

ncase=1, Table 2.1

t	z	u2(z,t)
1.0	0.0	6.062e-02
1.0	5.0	4.845e-02

```
1.0   10.0    4.100e-02
1.0   15.0    3.328e-02
1.0   20.0    2.319e-02
```

ncase=2, Table 2.2

```
 t      z      u2(z,t)
1.0    0.0    4.991e-02
1.0    5.0    3.417e-02
1.0   10.0    1.704e-02
1.0   15.0    2.524e-03
1.0   20.0    1.833e-04
```

This reduction for ncase=2 is also confirmed by comparing Figs. 2.1-3,4 with Figs. 2.2-3,4 (that follow). $u_2(z,t)$ remains low (after IC (1.2-2)) near $z = z_u = 20$.

- The secondary protein concentration is lower for ncase=2 than for ncase=1 (except at $z = 0.5$) from the exhalation for ncase=2.

ncase=1, Table 2.1

```
 t      z      u3(z,t)
1.0    0.0    3.451e-02
1.0    5.0    1.908e-02
1.0   10.0    1.279e-02
1.0   15.0    8.034e-03
1.0   20.0    4.063e-03
```

ncase=2, Table 2.2

```
 t      z      u3(z,t)
1.0    0.0    3.175e-02
1.0    5.0    2.036e-02
1.0   10.0    1.054e-02
```

```
1.0   15.0    1.529e-03
1.0   20.0    5.716e-05
```

This reduction for ncase=2 is also confirmed by comparing Figs. 2.1-5,6 with Figs. 2.2-5,6 (that follow). $u_3(z,t)$ remains low (after IC (1.2-3)) near $z = z_u = 20$.

- The virion population is lower for ncase=2 than for ncase=1 (except at $z = z_l = 0$) as expected (from the exhalation for ncase=2).

ncase=1, Table 2.1

t	z	u4(z,t)
1.0	0.0	0.000e+00
1.0	5.0	4.344e-04
1.0	10.0	3.647e-04
1.0	15.0	2.381e-04
1.0	20.0	1.101e-04

ncase=2, Table 2.2

t	z	u4(z,t)
1.0	0.0	6.207e-04
1.0	5.0	3.478e-04
1.0	10.0	1.346e-04
1.0	15.0	1.485e-05
1.0	20.0	1.146e-06

- The computational effort as indicated by ncall = 616 is modest so that lsodes computed the solution to eqs. (1.1), (1.2), (1.3) efficiently.

The graphical output is in Figs. 2.2.

The solution $u_1(z,t)$ starts from IC (1.2-1), and reflects BC (1.3-1) (at $z = z_l = 0$). The solution $u_1(z = z_l = 0, t)$ is not included as discussed previously.

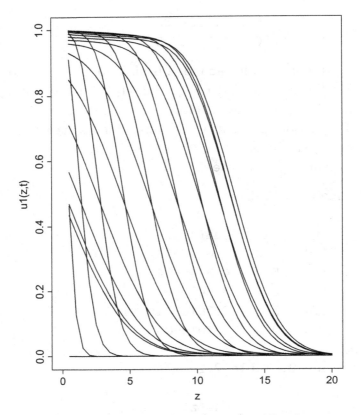

Figure 2.2-1: $u_1(z,t)$ from eq. (1.1-1), 2D from `matplot`, `ncase=2`

The solution $u_1(z,t)$ starts from IC (1.2-1), and reflects BC (1.3-1) (at $z = z_l = 0$). $u_1(z = z_l = 0, t)$ is included in the figure.

The solution $u_2(z,t)$ starts from IC (1.2-2), and reflects the response to BC (1.3-1) (at $z = z_l = 0$). The solution $u_2(z = z_l = 0, t)$ is not included as discussed previously.

The solutions in Figs. 1.2-3,4 reflect the invasion of the VGM into the host cells.

The solution $u_3(z,t)$ starts from IC (1.2-3), and indicates the production of the secondary protein within the host cells.

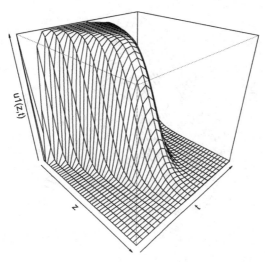

Figure 2.2-2: $u_1(z,t)$ from eq. (1.1-1), 3D from `persp`, `ncase=2`

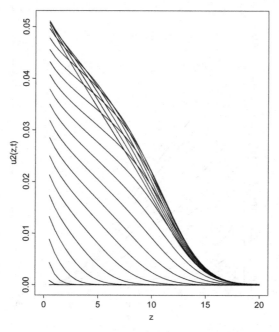

Figure 2.2-3: $u_2(z,t)$ from eq. (1.1-2), 2D from `matplot`, `ncase=2`

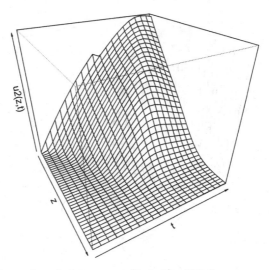

Figure 2.2-4: $u_2(z,t)$ from eq. (1.1-1), 3D from `persp`, `ncase=2`

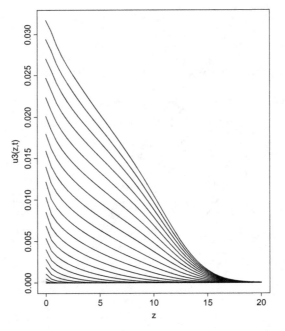

Figure 2.2-5: $u_3(z,t)$ from eq. (1.1-3), 2D from `matplot`, `ncase=2`

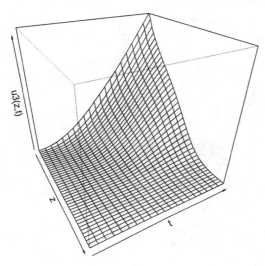

Figure 2.2-6: $u_3(z,t)$ from eq. (1.1-3), 3D from `persp`, ncase=2

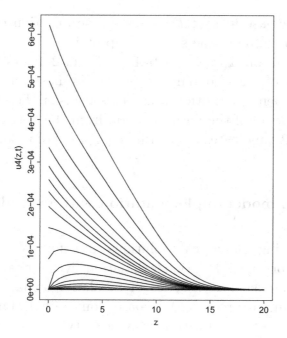

Figure 2.2-7: $u_4(z,t)$ from eq. (1.1-4), 2D from `matplot`, ncase=2

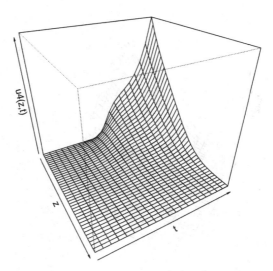

Figure 2.2-8: $u_4(z,t)$ from eq. (1.1-4), 3D from `persp`

The increase in $u_3(z,t)$ indicates the infection of the host cells by producton of the secondary protein.

The solution $u_4(z,t)$ starts from IC (1.2-4), and indicates the transfer of the secondary protein out of host cells as virions which can then infect other cells. This transfer therefore represents the spread of the viral infection from the host cells.

Fig. 2.2-8 indicates the continuing spread of virions to other host cells.

(2.2) PDE model implementation with extended time scale

The preceding numerical solutions are for one inhalation (`ncase=1`) or one inhalation/exhalation cycle (`ncase=2`). The following extension to a series of inhalation/exhalation cycles (to approximate breathing) is based on a final time increase from $t_f = 1$ to $t_f = 10$ with airway velocity $v_1 = 40\sin(2\pi t)$

(2.2.1) Main program

The following main program is a variant of the main program of Listing 2.1.

```
#
# Four PDE model
#
# Delete previous workspaces
  rm(list=ls(all=TRUE))
#
# Access ODE integrator
  library("deSolve");
#
# Access functions for numerical solution
  setwd("f:/chap2");
  source("pde1b.R");
#
# Parameters
  u1e=1;
  r2=1;
  n2=1;
  ke12=1;
  ke34=1;
  km12=0.1;
  km34=0.1;
  u10=0;
  u20=0;
  u30=0;
  u40=0;
#
# Spatial grid (in z)
  nz=41;zl=0;zu=20;dz=(zu-zl)/(nz-1)
  z=seq(from=zl,to=zu,by=dz);
#
```

```
# Independent variable for ODE integration
  t0=0;tf=10;nout=101;
  tout=seq(from=t0,to=tf,by=(tf-t0)/(nout-1));
#
# Initial condition (t=0)
  u0=rep(0,4*nz);
  for(i in 1:nz){
    u0[i]      =u10;
    u0[i+nz]   =u20;
    u0[i+2*nz]=u30;
    u0[i+3*nz]=u40;
  }
  ncall=0;
#
# ODE integration
  out=lsodes(y=u0,times=tout,func=pde1b,
      sparsetype ="sparseint",rtol=1e-6,
      atol=1e-6,maxord=5);
  nrow(out)
  ncol(out)
#
# Arrays for plotting numerical solution
  u1=matrix(0,nrow=nz,ncol=nout);
  u2=matrix(0,nrow=nz,ncol=nout);
  u3=matrix(0,nrow=nz,ncol=nout);
  u4=matrix(0,nrow=nz,ncol=nout);
  for(it in 1:nout){
    for(i in 1:nz){
      u1[i,it]=out[it,i+1];
      u2[i,it]=out[it,i+1+nz];
      u3[i,it]=out[it,i+1+2*nz];
      u4[i,it]=out[it,i+1+3*nz];
    }
  }
```

```
#
# Display numerical solution
  iv=seq(from=1,to=nout,by=50);
  for(it in iv){
    v1=40*sin(2*pi*tout[it]);
    if(v1>=0){
      u1[1,it]=u1e;
      u4[1,it]=0;}
    cat(sprintf("\n t = %6.2f v1 = %6.2f\n",
      tout[it],v1));
    cat(sprintf("\n     t     z       u1(z,t)\n"));
    iv=seq(from=1,to=nz,by=10);
    for(i in iv){
      cat(sprintf("%6.1f%6.1f%12.3e\n",
          tout[it],z[i],u1[i,it]));
    }
    cat(sprintf("\n     t     z       u2(z,t)\n"));
    iv=seq(from=1,to=nz,by=10);
    for(i in iv){
      cat(sprintf("%6.1f%6.1f%12.3e\n",
          tout[it],z[i],u2[i,it]));
    }
    cat(sprintf("\n     t     z       u3(z,t)\n"));
    iv=seq(from=1,to=nz,by=10);
    for(i in iv){
      cat(sprintf("%6.1f%6.1f%12.3e\n",
          tout[it],z[i],u3[i,it]));
    }
    cat(sprintf("\n     t     z       u4(z,t)\n"));
    iv=seq(from=1,to=nz,by=10);
    for(i in iv){
      cat(sprintf("%6.1f%6.1f%12.3e\n",
          tout[it],z[i],u4[i,it]));
    }
```

```
  }
#
# Calls to ODE routine
  cat(sprintf("\n\n ncall = %5d\n\n",ncall));
#
# Plot PDE solutions
#
# u1(z,t)
# 2D
  par(mfrow=c(1,1));
# matplot(x=z[2:nz],y=u1[2:nz,],type="l",xlab="z",
#   ylab="u1(z,t)",xlim=c(zl,zu),lty=1,main="",
#   lwd=2,col="black");
#
# 3D
  persp(z[2:nz],tout,u1[2:nz,],theta=45,phi=30,
        xlim=c(zl,zu),ylim=c(t0,tf),xlab="z",
        ylab="t",zlab="u1(,t)");
#
# u2(z,t)
# 2D
# par(mfrow=c(1,1));
# matplot(x=z[2:nz],y=u2[2:nz,],type="l",xlab="z",
#   ylab="u2(z,t)",xlim=c(zl,zu),lty=1,main="",
#   lwd=2,col="black");
#
# 3D
  persp(z[2:nz],tout,u2[2:nz,],theta=60,phi=30,
        xlim=c(zl,zu),ylim=c(t0,tf),xlab="z",
        ylab="t",zlab="u2(,t)");
#
# u3(z,t)
# 2D
# par(mfrow=c(1,1));
```

```
#   matplot(x=z,y=u3,type="l",xlab="z",
#     ylab="u3(z,t)",xlim=c(zl,zu),lty=1,
#     main="",lwd=2,col="black");
#
# 3D
  persp(z[2:nz],tout,u3[2:nz,],theta=60,phi=30,
        xlim=c(zl,zu),ylim=c(t0,tf),xlab="z",
        ylab="t",zlab="u3(,t)");
#
# u4(z,t)
# 2D
# par(mfrow=c(1,1));
# matplot(x=z,y=u4,type="l",xlab="z",
#     ylab="u4(z,t)",xlim=c(zl,zu),lty=1,
#     main="",lwd=2,col="black");
#
# 3D
  persp(z[2:nz],tout,u4[2:nz,],theta=60,phi=30,
        xlim=c(zl,zu),ylim=c(t0,tf),xlab="z",
        ylab="t",zlab="u4(,t)");
#
# Plot v1(t)
  v1p=rep(0,nout);
  for(it in 1:nout){
    v1p[it]=40*sin(2*pi*tout[it]);}
  par(mfrow=c(1,1));
  plot(x=tout,y=v1p,type="l",xlab="t (sec)",
    ylab="v1(t)",xlim=c(t0,tf),lty=1,main="",
    lwd=2,col="black");
```

Listing 2.3: Main program for eqs. (1.1), (1.2), (1.3) $t_f = 10$

We can note the following details of Listing 2.3 for $t_f = 10$, particularly the changes in Listing 2.1.

- The ODE/MOL routine is pde1b.

```
#
# Access functions for numerical solution
  setwd("f:/chap2");
  source("pde1b.R");
```

- The parameters of Listing 2.1 are repeated here.

```
#
# Parameters
  u1e=1;
  r2=1;
  n2=1;
  ke12=1;
  ke34=1;
  km12=0.1;
  km34=0.1;
  u10=0;
  u20=0;
  u30=0;
  u40=0;
```

- The time scale is expanded to $t_f = 10$ with 101 output points.

```
#
# Independent variable for ODE integration
  t0=0;tf=10;nout=101;
  tout=seq(from=t0,to=tf,by=(tf-t0)/(nout-1));
```

- lsodes calls pde1b.

```
#
# ODE integration
  out=lsodes(y=u0,times=tout,func=pde1b,
      sparsetype ="sparseint",rtol=1e-6,
```

```
      atol=1e-6,maxord=5);
   nrow(out)
   ncol(out)
```

- The airway linear velocity is $v_1(t) = 40\sin(2\pi t)$ (used in eqs. (1.1-1,4)).

```
#
# Display numerical solution
   iv=seq(from=1,to=nout,by=50);
   for(it in iv){
     v1=40*sin(2*pi*tout[it]);
```

Every 50th value in t is displayed with by=50.

- The PDE solutions, $u_1(z,t), u_2(z,t), u_3(z,t), u_4(z,t)$, are complicated when plotted in 2D by matplot, that is, parametrically in t with 101 curves. Therefore, the calls to matplot are commented. For example, for $u_1(z,t)$,

```
#
# Plot PDE solutions
#
# u1(z,t)
# 2D
   par(mfrow=c(1,1));
# matplot(x=z[2:nz],y=u1[2:nz,],type="l",xlab="z",
#    ylab="u1(z,t)",xlim=c(zl,zu),lty=1,main="",
#    lwd=2,col="black");
#
# 3D
   persp(z[2:nz],tout,u1[2:nz,],theta=45,phi=30,
        xlim=c(zl,zu),ylim=c(t0,tf),xlab="z",
        ylab="t",zlab="u1(,t)");
```

The 3D plotting from persp does not include the solution at $z = z_l = 0$ because of the discontinuity between the IC (eq. (1.2-1)), $u_1(z = 0, t = 0) = 0$, and BC (1.3-1), $u_1(z = 0, t > 0) = u_{1e} = $ `u1e=1`. That is, `z[2:nz],u1[2:nz,]` are used.

The use of `matplot` (by uncommenting) and `persp` with $z = z_l = 0$ are left as exercises.

- The calls to `matplot`, `persp` for $u_2(z,t), u_3(z,t), u_4(z,t)$ are modified in the same way as for $u_1(z,t)$.

```
#
# u2(z,t)
# 2D
# par(mfrow=c(1,1));
# matplot(x=z[2:nz],y=u2[2:nz,],type="l",xlab="z",
#   ylab="u2(z,t)",xlim=c(zl,zu),lty=1,main="",
#   lwd=2,col="black");
#
# 3D
  persp(z[2:nz],tout,u2[2:nz,],theta=60,phi=30,
        xlim=c(zl,zu),ylim=c(t0,tf),xlab="z",
        ylab="t",zlab="u2(,t)");
#
# u3(z,t)
# 2D
# par(mfrow=c(1,1));
#  matplot(x=z,y=u3,type="l",xlab="z",
#     ylab="u3(z,t)",xlim=c(zl,zu),lty=1,
#     main="",lwd=2,col="black");
#
# 3D
  persp(z[2:nz],tout,u3[2:nz,],theta=60,phi=30,
        xlim=c(zl,zu),ylim=c(t0,tf),xlab="z",
        ylab="t",zlab="u3(,t)");
#
# u4(z,t)
```

```
# 2D
# par(mfrow=c(1,1));
# matplot(x=z,y=u4,type="l",xlab="z",
#   ylab="u4(z,t)",xlim=c(zl,zu),lty=1,
#   main="",lwd=2,col="black");
#
# 3D
  persp(z[2:nz],tout,u4[2:nz,],theta=60,phi=30,
        xlim=c(zl,zu),ylim=c(t0,tf),xlab="z",
        ylab="t",zlab="u4(,t)");
```

- The velocity $v_1(t)$ is plotted with `plot`.

```
#
# Plot v1(t)
  v1p=rep(0,nout);
  for(it in 1:nout){
    v1p[it]=40*sin(2*pi*tout[it]);}
  par(mfrow=c(1,1));
  plot(x=tout,y=v1p,type="l",xlab="t (sec)",
    ylab="v1(t)",xlim=c(t0,tf),lty=1,main="",
    lwd=2,col="black");
```

This completes the discussion of the main program in Listing 2.3. The ODE/MOL routine `pde1b` is considered next.

(2.2.2) ODE/MOL routine

`pde1b` is the same as `pde1a` of Listing 2.2 except for the programming of the velocity $v_1(t)$ (used in eqs. (1.1-1,4)).

```
  pde1a, Listing 2.2
#
# v1(t) for ncase=1,2
  if(ncase==1){
    v1=40*sin(  pi*(t-t0)/(tf-t0));}
```

```
if(ncase==2){
  v1=40*sin(2*pi*(t-t0)/(tf-t0));}
```

```
  pde1b
#
# v1(t)
  v1=40*sin(2*pi*t);
```

(2.2.3) Numerical, graphical output

The numerical output from the main program of Listing 2.3 (which calls pde1b) follows.

```
[1] 101
```

```
[1] 165
```

```
t =    0.00 v1 =    0.00
```

t	z	u1(z,t)
0.0	0.0	1.000e+00
0.0	5.0	0.000e+00
0.0	10.0	0.000e+00
0.0	15.0	0.000e+00
0.0	20.0	0.000e+00

t	z	u2(z,t)
0.0	0.0	0.000e+00
0.0	5.0	0.000e+00
0.0	10.0	0.000e+00
0.0	15.0	0.000e+00
0.0	20.0	0.000e+00

t	z	u3(z,t)
0.0	0.0	0.000e+00

```
0.0    5.0   0.000e+00
0.0   10.0   0.000e+00
0.0   15.0   0.000e+00
0.0   20.0   0.000e+00


  t      z      u4(z,t)
0.0    0.0   0.000e+00
0.0    5.0   0.000e+00
0.0   10.0   0.000e+00
0.0   15.0   0.000e+00
0.0   20.0   0.000e+00


t =    5.00 v1 =   -0.00


  t      z      u1(z,t)
5.0    0.0   6.852e-01
5.0    5.0   3.641e-01
5.0   10.0   2.434e-01
5.0   15.0   2.371e-01
5.0   20.0   2.371e-01


  t      z      u2(z,t)
5.0    0.0   8.152e-02
5.0    5.0   6.447e-02
5.0   10.0   4.380e-02
5.0   15.0   2.496e-02
5.0   20.0   1.785e-02


  t      z      u3(z,t)
5.0    0.0   2.767e-01
5.0    5.0   2.043e-01
5.0   10.0   1.251e-01
5.0   15.0   5.193e-02
5.0   20.0   2.820e-02
```

```
  t      z      u4(z,t)
 5.0    0.0    1.848e-02
 5.0    5.0    1.774e-02
 5.0   10.0    1.427e-02
 5.0   15.0    1.284e-02
 5.0   20.0    1.256e-02
```

t =   10.00 v1 =   -0.00

```
  t      z      u1(z,t)
10.0    0.0    7.372e-01
10.0    5.0    4.905e-01
10.0   10.0    4.000e-01
10.0   15.0    3.953e-01
10.0   20.0    3.952e-01
```

```
  t      z      u2(z,t)
10.0    0.0    8.339e-02
10.0    5.0    7.027e-02
10.0   10.0    5.451e-02
10.0   15.0    4.022e-02
10.0   20.0    3.486e-02
```

```
  t      z      u3(z,t)
10.0    0.0    5.060e-01
10.0    5.0    4.061e-01
10.0   10.0    2.914e-01
10.0   15.0    1.843e-01
10.0   20.0    1.444e-01
```

```
  t      z      u4(z,t)
10.0    0.0    5.329e-02
10.0    5.0    7.081e-02
```

```
10.0   10.0   7.084e-02
10.0   15.0   6.882e-02
10.0   20.0   6.834e-02

ncall =   3844
```

Table 2.3: Numerical output from Listings 2.3, 2.4

We can note the following details about this output (with some repetition of the discussion of Tables 2.1, 2.2 so that the following discussion is self contained).

- 101 t output points as the first dimension of the solution matrix out from lsodes as programmed in the main program of Listing 2.3 (with nout=101).
- The solution matrix out returned by lsodes has 165 elements as a second dimension. The first element is the value of t. Elements 2 to 165 are $u_1(z,t)$, $u_2(z,t)$, $u_3(z,t)$, $u_4(z,t)$ $(4(41) = 164$ points in z).
- The solution is displayed for t=0,10/100,...,10 as programmed in Listing 2.3 (every 50th value of t is displayed as explained previously).
- ICs (1.2) are confirmed $(t = 0)$. BC (1.3-1) is also confirmed reflecting the discontinuous change from the IC as discussed previously.

```
    t        z      u1(z,t)
   0.0      0.0    1.000e+00
```

- The increase in the secondary protein produced in the host cells is confirmed, e.g.,

```
    t        z      u3(z,t)
   10.0     0.0    5.060e-01
   10.0     5.0    4.061e-01
   10.0    10.0    2.914e-01
   10.0    15.0    1.843e-01
   10.0    20.0    1.444e-01
```

- The increase in the virion population exiting the host cells is confirmed, e.g.,

```
   t      z       u4(z,t)
 10.0    0.0     5.329e-02
 10.0    5.0     7.081e-02
 10.0   10.0     7.084e-02
 10.0   15.0     6.882e-02
 10.0   20.0     6.834e-02
```

These values are larger than for $t_f = 1$ (Table 2.2).
- The computational effort as indicated by `ncall` = 3844 reflects the increase of t_f from 1 (`ncall` =616, Table 2.2) to 10

The graphical oputput is in Figs. 2.3.

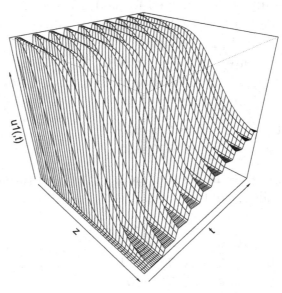

Figure 2.3-1: $u_1(z,t)$ from eq. (1.1-1), 3D from `persp`, $t_f = 10$

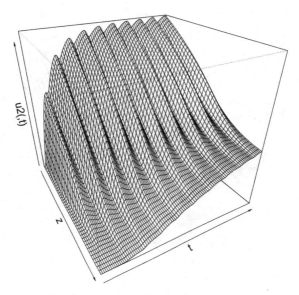

Figure 2.3-2: $u_2(z, t)$ from eq. (1.1-2), 3D from **persp**, $t_f = 10$

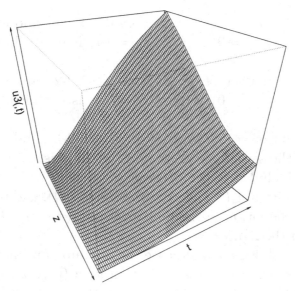

Figure 2.3-3: $u_3(z, t)$ from eq. (1.1-3), 3D from **persp**, $t_f = 10$

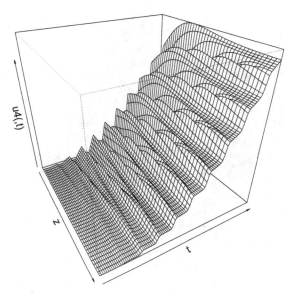

Figure 2.3-4: $u_4(z, t)$ from eq. (1.1-4), 3D from `persp`, $t_f = 10$

The solution $u_1(z, t)$ starts from IC (1.2-1), and reflects BC (1.3-1) (at $z = z_l = 0$). $u_1(z = z_l = 0, t)$ is not included in the figure.

The solution $u_2(z, t)$ starts from IC (1.2-2), and reflects BC (1.3-1) (at $z = z_l = 0$). $u_2(z = z_l = 0, t)$ is not included in the figure.

The solution $u_3(z, t)$ starts from IC (1.2-3), and reflects the buildup of the secondary protein in the lung tissue. $u_3(z = z_l = 0, t)$ is not included in the figure.

The solution $u_4(z, t)$ starts from IC (1.2-4), and reflects the buildup of the virion in the lung airway. $u_4(z = z_l = 0, t)$ is not included in the figure.

In general, Figs. 2.3 indicate the buildup of primary protein ($u_2(z, t)$, Fig. 2.3-2) and secondary protein ($u_3(z, t)$, Fig. 2.3-3) in the lung tissue (note, for example, the increasing values at $z = z_u$). Also, the increase in the virions with t is clear in Fig. 2.3-4.

(2.3) Summary and conclusions

The 4×4 (four equations in four unknowns) PDE model for the lung/respiratory system has been developed and explained. In general, the invasion of the virus into the lung tissue, and the production of virions that can further infect lung tissue is a principal output of the PDE model.

The model can now be used to study the treatment of an infected lung. For example, the postulated effect of a ventilator can be studied by including a reduction in the virus concentration, $u_1(a, t)$ of eq. (1.1-1), and the virion concentration, $u_4(z, t)$ of eq. (1.1-4).

References

[1] Schiesser, W.E. (2016), *Method of Lines Analysis in Biomedical Science and Engineering*, John Wiley, Hoboken, NJ, USA

[2] Soetaert, K., J. Cash, and F. Mazzia (2012), *Solving Differential Equations in R*, Springer-Verlag, Heidelberg, Germany.

Chapter 3
SVIR Model Formulation

(3) Introduction

A SVIR (**S**usceptible-**V**accinated-**I**nfected-**R**ecovered) model is formulated in this chapter as a system of ordinary differential equations (ODEs) in time, then extended to a system of partial differential equations (PDEs) to account for spatial effects (spatiotemporal modeling).

(3.1) ODE SVIR model formulation

The ODE SVIR model is based on population balances in time. The balance for susceptibles, with population density $\tilde{S}(t)$ is [1]

$$\frac{d\tilde{S}}{d\tilde{t}} = (1 - \epsilon)\Pi + \tilde{\omega}\tilde{V} + \tilde{\delta}\tilde{R} - \tilde{\beta}\tilde{S}\tilde{I} - \tilde{\xi}\tilde{S} - \mu\tilde{S} \qquad (3.1\text{-}1)$$

The ODE dependent variables are defined in Table 3.1, and the parameters are defined in Table 3.2. The terms in eq. (3.1-1) are explained briefly by the parameters in Table 3.2.

Similarly, the balances for vaccinated, infected and recovered population densities $\tilde{V}(t)$, $\tilde{I}(t)$, $\tilde{R}(t)$ are [1]

$$\frac{d\tilde{V}}{d\tilde{t}} = \tilde{\xi}\tilde{S} - (1 - \sigma)\tilde{\beta}\tilde{V}\tilde{I} - (\tilde{\omega} + \mu)\tilde{V} \qquad (3.1\text{-}2)$$

$$\frac{d\tilde{I}}{d\tilde{t}} = \epsilon\Pi + \tilde{\beta}\tilde{S}\tilde{I} + (1-\sigma)\tilde{\beta}\tilde{V}\tilde{I} - (\tilde{\alpha}+\mu)\tilde{I} \qquad (3.1\text{-}3)$$

$$\frac{d\tilde{R}}{d\tilde{t}} = \tilde{\alpha}\tilde{I} - (\mu+\tilde{\delta})\tilde{R} \qquad (3.1\text{-}4)$$

The dependent and independent variables of eqs. (3.1) are defined in Table 3.1.

$\tilde{S}$ susceptible population

$\tilde{V}$ vaccinated population

$\tilde{I}$ infected population

$\tilde{R}$ recovered population

$\tilde{t}$ time

Table 3.1: ODE model variables

The parameters of eqs. (3.1) are defined in Table 3.2 [1], p507.

Π recruitment rate of individuals

ϵ fraction of recruited individuals who are infected

$\tilde{\beta}$ $\dfrac{\text{contacts}}{\text{time}} \times$ probability of infection per contact

with an infected individual

$\tilde{\xi}$ rate at which susceptible individuals are vaccinated

σ vaccine efficacy

$\tilde{\omega}$ rate at which vaccine-based immunity wanes

$1/\tilde{\omega}$ average time to lose vaccine-induced immunity

$\tilde{\alpha}$ recovery rate from infection

$1/\tilde{\alpha}$ average length of infection (duration of infectiousness)

$\tilde{\delta}$ rate of loss of immunity acquired by infection

$1/\tilde{\delta}$ average time to lose immunity acquired by infection

μ rate at which people leave the population
(assumed to be the same for the four populations)

$1/\mu$ average life-span

Table 3.2: ODE model parameters

The terms in eqs. (3.1) are explained briefly by the parameters in Table 3.2. A schematic diagram for eqs. (3.1) is given in [1], Fig. 2.

To facilitate the subsequent analytical and numerical analysis of the ODE model of eqs. (3.1), normalized variables and parameters are defined.

$$S = \frac{\mu}{\Pi}\tilde{S}, \ V = \frac{\mu}{\Pi}\tilde{V}, \ I = \frac{\mu}{\Pi}\tilde{I}, \ R = \frac{\mu}{\Pi}\tilde{R} \qquad (3.2\text{-}1)$$

$$t = \mu\tilde{t}, \ \beta = \frac{\Pi\tilde{\beta}}{\mu^2}, \ \omega = \frac{\tilde{\omega}}{\mu}, \ \xi = \frac{\tilde{\xi}}{\mu}, \ \delta = \frac{\tilde{\delta}}{\mu}, \ \delta = \frac{\tilde{\delta}}{\mu}, \ \alpha = \frac{\tilde{\alpha}}{\mu}$$
$$(3.2\text{-}2)$$

Substitution of the normalized variables and parameters in eq. (3.1-1) gives

$$\frac{d(\Pi/\mu)S}{dt/\mu} = (1 - \epsilon)\Pi + (\mu\omega)(\Pi/\mu)V + (\mu\delta)(\Pi/\mu)R$$

$$-(\mu^2/\Pi)\beta(\Pi/\mu)S(\Pi/\mu)I - (\mu\xi)(\Pi/\mu)S - \mu(\Pi/\mu)S$$

or

$$\frac{dS}{dt} = (1 - \epsilon) + \omega V + \delta R - \beta SI - \xi S - S \qquad (3.3\text{-}1)$$

Eq. (3.3-1) for the normalized susceptible population density, $S(t)$, is the first ODE of the 4×4 (four equations in four unknowns) ODE model. The derivation of the ODEs for the normalized variables $V(t)$, $I(t)$, $R(t)$ follows in the same way [1].

$$\frac{dV}{dt} = \xi S - (1 - \sigma)\beta VI - (1 + \omega)V \qquad (3.3\text{-}2)$$

$$\frac{dI}{dt} = \epsilon + \beta SI + (1 - \sigma)\beta VI - (1 + \alpha)I \qquad (3.3\text{-}3)$$

$$\frac{dR}{dt} = \alpha I - (1 + \delta)R \qquad (3.3\text{-}4)$$

A feature of the ODE model can be observed by adding eqs. (3.3).

$$\frac{dS}{dt} + \frac{dV}{dt} + \frac{dI}{dt} + \frac{dR}{dt} = 1 - (S + V + I + R)$$

or with $N(t) = S(t) + V(t) + I(t) + R(t)$, the ODE for the total population $N(t)$ is

$$\frac{dN}{dt} = 1 - N \qquad (3.3\text{-}5)$$

With N(t=0)=1, eq. has the solution $N(t) = 1$.

(3.2) PDE SVIR model formulation

Eqs. (3.3) do not account for spatial effects in defining the dynamic aspects of $S(t), V(t), I(t), R(t)$. To include spatial effects, diffusion terms are added to eqs. (3.3). For example, eq. (3.3-1) is

$$\frac{\partial S}{\partial t} = D_S(\frac{\partial^2 S}{\partial r^2} + \frac{1}{r}\frac{\partial S}{\partial r}) + (1 - \epsilon) + \omega V + \delta R - \beta SI - \xi S - S$$

$$(3.4\text{-}1)$$

where r is the radial coordinate in polar coordinates, (r, θ), or cylindrical coordinates (r, θ, z). The spatial dispersion of the susceptibles is modeled as linear (Fickian) diffusion, $D_S(\frac{\partial^2 S}{\partial r^2} + \frac{1}{r}\frac{\partial S}{\partial r})$ where D_S is a diffusivity for self diffusion of $S(t)$.

Similarly, ODEs (3.3-2,3,4) are extended to PDEs (3.4-2,3,4).

$$\frac{\partial V}{\partial t} = D_V \left(\frac{\partial^2 V}{\partial r^2} + \frac{1}{r}\frac{\partial V}{\partial r}\right) + \xi S - (1-\sigma)\beta VI - (1+\omega)V \quad (3.4\text{-}2)$$

$$\frac{\partial I}{\partial t} = D_I \left(\frac{\partial^2 I}{\partial r^2} + \frac{1}{r}\frac{\partial I}{\partial r}\right) + \epsilon + \beta SI + (1-\sigma)\beta VI - (1+\alpha)I \quad (3.4\text{-}3)$$

$$\frac{\partial R}{\partial t} = D_R \left(\frac{\partial^2 R}{\partial r^2} + \frac{1}{r}\frac{\partial R}{\partial r}\right) + \alpha I - (1+\delta)R \quad (3.4\text{-}4)$$

The ODE system, eqs. (3.3), is first order in t so that each equation requires an initial condition (IC).

$$S(t = 0) = S_0; \; V(t = 0) = V_0; \; I(t = 0) = I_0; \; R(t = 0) = R_0$$

$$(3.5\text{-}1,2,3,4)$$

Similarly, the PDE system, eqs. (3.4), is first order in t so that each equation requires an initial condition (IC).

$$S(t = 0) = S_0(r); \; V(t = 0) = V_0(r);$$
$$I(t = 0) = I_0(r); \; R(t = 0) = R_0(r)$$

$$(3.6\text{-}1,2,3,4)$$

The PDE system, eqs. (3.4), is second order in r so that each equation requires two boundary conditions (BCs). At $r = r_l = 0$, the BCs are

$$\frac{\partial S(r = r_l = 0, t)}{\partial r} = 0 \qquad (3.7\text{-}1)$$

$$\frac{\partial V(r = r_l = 0, t)}{\partial r} = 0 \qquad (3.7\text{-}2)$$

$$\frac{\partial I(r = r_l = 0, t)}{\partial r} = 0 \qquad (3.7\text{-}3)$$

$$\frac{\partial R(r = r_l = 0, t)}{\partial r} = 0 \qquad (3.7\text{-}4)$$

BCs (3.7) specify symmetry (and zero flux) at $r = r_l = 0$.
At $r = r_u$, the BC for eq. (3.4-1) is

$$D_S \frac{\partial S(r = r_u, t)}{\partial r} = k_s(S_b - S(r = r_u, t)) \qquad (3.8\text{-}1)$$

This BC equates the diffusion flux of $S(r = r_l, t)$ to the transfer
flux resulting from an ambient susceptibles denslty, S_b.

Eqs. (3.7-1), (3.8-1) are the two BCs for eq. (3.4-1).
Similarly, eqs. (3.7-2), (3.8-2) are the two BCs for eq. (3.4-2)

$$\frac{\partial V(r = r_u, t)}{\partial r} = \frac{1}{D_V} k_v(V_b - V(r = r_u, t)) \qquad (3.8\text{-}2)$$

Eqs. (3.7-3), (3.8-3) are the BCs for eq. (3.4-3).

$$\frac{\partial I(r = r_u, t)}{\partial r} = \frac{1}{D_I} k_i(I_b - I(r = r_u, t)) \qquad (3.8\text{-}3)$$

Eqs. (3.7-4), (3.8-4) are the BCs for eq. (3.4-4).

$$\frac{\partial R(r = r_u, t)}{\partial r} = \frac{1}{D_R} k_R(R_b - R(r = r_u, t)) \qquad (3.8\text{-}4)$$

This completes the formulation of the PDE model.

(3.3) Summary and conclusions

The SVIR model discussed in this chapter has two variants:

- An ODE model for which the dependent variables $S(t), V(t), I(t), R(t)$ are functions of time t, as defined by eqs. (3.3) and ICs (3.5).
- A PDE model which accounts for time and space to give spatiotemporal solutions, $S(r, t), V(r, t), I(r, t), R(r, t)$ as defined by eqs. (3.4), ICs (3.6), and BCs (3.7) and (3.8).

These two models are implemented in a series of R routines as explained in the next chapter.

References

[1] Alexander, M.E., et al (2004), A Vaccination Model for Transmission Dynamics of Influenza, *SIAM Journal Applied Dynamical Systems*, **3**, no. 3, pp 503-524

Appendix A3: Derivation of the four PDE model

The derivation of the $S(r, t)$ PDE, eq. (3.4-1), is based on a susceptibles population balance for an incremental volume $2\pi r \Delta r \Delta z$.

$$2\pi r \Delta r \Delta z \frac{\partial S(r, t)}{\partial t} =$$

$$D_S \left(-2\pi r \Delta z \frac{\partial S(r, t)}{\partial r} \right) \Big|_{r - \Delta r}$$

$$-D_S \left(-2\pi r \Delta z \frac{\partial S(r, t)}{\partial r} \right) \Big|_r$$

$$+2\pi r \Delta r \Delta z (\omega V(r, t) + \delta R(r, t) - \beta S(r, t) I(r, t) - \xi S(r, t) - S(r, t))$$

$$(A3.1)$$

An explanation of the terms in eq. (A3.1) follows.

- $2\pi r \Delta r \Delta z \dfrac{\partial S(r,t)}{\partial t}$: Rate of accumulation (term is positive) or depletion (term is negative) of susceptibles in the incremental volume $2\pi r \Delta r \Delta z$.

- $D_S\left(-2\pi r \Delta z \dfrac{\partial S(r,t)}{\partial r}\right)|_{r-\Delta r}$: Rate of self diffusion through the incremental area $2\pi r \Delta z$ at $r - \Delta r$.

- $D_S\left(-2\pi r \Delta z \dfrac{\partial S(r,t)}{\partial r}\right)|_{r}$: Rate of self diffusion through the incremental area $2\pi r \Delta z$ at r.

- $2\pi r \Delta r \Delta z (\omega V(r,t) + \delta R(r,t) - \beta S(r,t) I(r,t) - \xi S(r,t) - S(r,t))$: Rate of change of susceptibles in the incremental volume $2\pi r \Delta r \Delta z$.

Division of eq. (A3.1) by $2\pi r \Delta r \Delta z$ and rearrangement gives

$$\frac{\partial S(r,t)}{\partial t} =$$

$$\frac{D_S}{r}\left(\frac{r\dfrac{\partial S(r,t)}{\partial r}\Big|_{r} - r\dfrac{\partial S(r,t)}{\partial r}\Big|_{r-\Delta r}}{\Delta r}\right)$$

$$+\omega V(r,t) + \delta R(r,t) - \beta S(r,t) I(r,t) - \xi S(r,t) - S(r,t) \quad \text{(A3.2)}$$

With $\Delta r \to 0$, eq. (A3.2) is

$$\frac{\partial S(r,t)}{\partial t} =$$

$$\frac{D_S}{r}\frac{\partial\left(r\dfrac{\partial S(r,t)}{\partial r}\right)}{\partial r}$$

$$+\omega V(r,t) + \delta R(r,t) - \beta S(r,t) I(r,t) - \xi S(r,t) - S(r,t) \quad \text{(A3.3)}$$

Expansion of the radial term in eq. (A3.3) gives

$$\frac{\partial S(r,t)}{\partial t} =$$

$$D_S \left(\frac{\partial^2 S(r,t)}{\partial r^2} + \frac{1}{r} \frac{\partial S(r,t)}{\partial r} \right)$$

$$+\omega V(r,t) + \delta R(r,t) - \beta S(r,t) I(r,t) - \xi S(r,t) - S(r,t) \quad \text{(A3.4)}$$

Eq. (A3.4) is eq. (3.4-1).

An analogous development for the vaccinated, infected and recovered populations, $V(r,t), I(r,t), R(r,t)$, leads to eqs. (3.4-2,3,4).

Chapter 4

SVIR Model Implementation

(4) Introduction

The SVIR ODE and PDE models formulated in Chapter 3 are implemented in R as explained in this chapter.

(4.1) ODE model implementation

A main program for the ODE model of eqs. (3.3) with ICs (3.5) follows.

(4.1.1) Main program

```
#
# Four ODE model
#
# Delete previous workspaces
  rm(list=ls(all=TRUE))
#
# Access ODE integrator
  library("deSolve");
#
# Access functions for numerical solution
  setwd("f:/chap4");
  source("ode1a.R");
#
```

```
# Parameters
  alpha=0.25;
  beta=4.5;
  delta=1;
  eps=0.25;
  xi=10;
  omega=1;
  sigma=0.2;
  ne=4;
#
# Independent variable for ODE integration
  t0=0;tf=2;nout=21;
  tout=seq(from=t0,to=tf,by=(tf-t0)/(nout-1));
#
# Initial condition (t=0)
  u0=rep(0,ne);
  u0[1]=1;
  ncall=0;
#
# ODE integration
  out=lsodes(y=u0,times=tout,func=ode1a,
      sparsetype ="sparseint",rtol=1e-6,
      atol=1e-6,maxord=5);
  nrow(out)
  ncol(out)
#
# Arrays for plotting numerical solution
  t=rep(0,nout);
  S=rep(0,nout);
  V=rep(0,nout);
  I=rep(0,nout);
  R=rep(0,nout);
  for(it in 1:nout){
    t[it]=out[it,1];
```

```
    S[it]=out[it,2];
    V[it]=out[it,3];
    I[it]=out[it,4];
    R[it]=out[it,5];
  }
#
# Display numerical solution
  iv=seq(from=1,to=nout,by=5);
  for(it in iv){
    cat(sprintf("\n\n  t = %6.2f   S = %6.3f",
        tout[it],S[it]));
    cat(sprintf("\n  t = %6.2f   V = %6.3f",
        tout[it],V[it]));
    cat(sprintf("\n  t = %6.2f   I = %6.3f",
        tout[it],I[it]));
    cat(sprintf("\n  t = %6.2f   R = %6.3f",
        tout[it],R[it]));
  }
#
# Calls to ODE routine
  cat(sprintf("\n\n ncall = %5d\n\n",ncall));
#
# Plot ODE solutions
#
# S(t)
  par(mfrow=c(2,2));
  matplot(x=t,y=S,type="l",xlab="t",
    ylab="S(t)",xlim=c(t0,tf),lty=1,
    main="",lwd=2,col="black");
#
# V(t)
  matplot(x=t,y=V,type="l",xlab="t",
    ylab="V(t)",xlim=c(t0,tf),lty=1,
    main="",lwd=2,col="black");
```

```
#
# I(t)
  matplot(x=t,y=I,type="l",xlab="t",
    ylab="I(t)",xlim=c(t0,tf),lty=1,
    main="",lwd=2,col="black");
#
# R(t)
  matplot(x=t,y=R,type="l",xlab="t",
    ylab="R(t)",xlim=c(t0,tf),lty=1,
    main="",lwd=2,col="black");
```

Listing 4.1: Main program for eqs. (3.3), (3.5)

We can note the following details about Listing 4.1.

- Previous workspaces are deleted.

  ```
  #
  #  Four ODE model
  #
  # Delete previous workspaces
    rm(list=ls(all=TRUE))
  ```

- The R ODE integrator library deSolve is accessed [2]. Then the directory with the files for the solution of eqs. (3.3) is designated. Note that setwd (set working directory) uses / rather than the usual \.

  ```
  #
  # Access ODE integrator
    library("deSolve");
  #
  # Access functions for numerical solution
    setwd("f:/chap4");
    source("ode1a.R");
  ```

ode1a is the ODE routine for eqs. (3.3), discussed subsequently.

- The model parameters are specified numerically.

```
#
# Parameters
  alpha=0.25;
  beta=4.5;
  delta=1;
  eps=0.25;
  xi=10;
  omega=1;
  sigma=0.2;
  ne=4;
```

The parameters are named in analogy with eqs. (3.3). For example, alpha = α in eqs. (3.3-3,4). Of particular interest is the low vaccine efficacy, sigma=0.2.

- An interval in t is defined for 21 output points, so that tout=0,2/20,...,2 (yr).

```
#
# Independent variable for ODE integration
  t0=0;tf=2;nout=21;
  tout=seq(from=t0,to=tf,by=(tf-t0)/(nout-1));
```

- ICs (3.5) are placed in a vector u0 of length ne=4.

```
#
# Initial condition (t=0)
  u0=rep(0,ne);
  u0[1]=1;
  ncall=0;
```

For this case, the ICs are $S(t = 0) = 1$, $V(t = 0) = I(t = 0) = R(t = 0) = 0$. Also, the counter for the calls to pde1a is initialized.

- The system of 4 ODEs is integrated by the library integrator `lsodes` (available in `deSolve`, [2]). As expected, the inputs to `lsodes` are the ODE function, `ode1a`, the IC vector u0, and the vector of output values of t, `tout`. The length of u0 (4) informs `lsodes` how many ODEs are to be integrated. `func,y,times` are reserved names.

```
#
# ODE integration
  out=lsodes(y=u0,times=tout,func=ode1a,
      sparsetype ="sparseint",rtol=1e-6,
      atol=1e-6,maxord=5);
  nrow(out)
  ncol(out)
```

nrow,ncol confirm the dimensions of out.

- $t, S(t), V(t), I(t), R(t)$ from matrix out returned by `lsodes` are placed in vectors for subsequent plotting.

```
#
# Arrays for plotting numerical solution
  t=rep(0,nout);
  S=rep(0,nout);
  V=rep(0,nout);
  I=rep(0,nout);
  R=rep(0,nout);
  for(it in 1:nout){
    t[it]=out[it,1];
    S[it]=out[it,2];
    V[it]=out[it,3];
    I[it]=out[it,4];
    R[it]=out[it,5];
  }
```

- The values of $t, S(t), V(t), I(t), R(t)$ are displayed as a function of t with a `for`.

```
#
# Display numerical solution
  iv=seq(from=1,to=nout,by=5);
  for(it in iv){
    cat(sprintf("\n\n t = %6.2f   S = %6.3f",
        tout[it],S[it]));
    cat(sprintf("\n t = %6.2f   V = %6.3f",
        tout[it],V[it]));
    cat(sprintf("\n t = %6.2f   I = %6.3f",
        tout[it],I[it]));
    cat(sprintf("\n t = %6.2f   R = %6.3f",
        tout[it],R[it]));
  }
```

Every fifth values of $S(t), V(t), I(t), R(t)$ are displayed by=5.

- The total number of calls to ode1a is displayed.

```
#
# Calls to ODE routine
  cat(sprintf("\n\n ncall = %5d\n\n",ncall));
```

- The solutions $S(t), V(t), I(t), R(t)$ are plotted in 2D with the utility matplot

```
#
# Plot ODE solutions
#
# S(t)
  par(mfrow=c(2,2));
  matplot(x=t,y=S,type="l",xlab="t",
    ylab="S(t)",xlim=c(t0,tf),lty=1,
    main="",lwd=2,col="black");
#
# V(t)
  matplot(x=t,y=V,type="l",xlab="t",
```

```
        ylab="V(t)",xlim=c(t0,tf),lty=1,
        main="",lwd=2,col="black");
  #
  # I(t)
      matplot(x=t,y=I,type="l",xlab="t",
        ylab="I(t)",xlim=c(t0,tf),lty=1,
        main="",lwd=2,col="black");
  #
  # R(t)
      matplot(x=t,y=R,type="l",xlab="t",
        ylab="R(t)",xlim=c(t0,tf),lty=1,
        main="",lwd=2,col="black");
```

This completes the discussion of the main program in Listing 4.1. The ODE routine called by `lsodes` in the main program is considered next.

(4.1.2) ODE routine

The ODE routine for eqs. (3.3) called by `lsodes` follows.

```
  ode1a=function(t,y,parm){
#
# Function pde1a computes the t derivatives
# of S(t),V(t),I(t),R(t)
#
# One vector to four scalars
  S=y[1];
  V=y[2];
  I=y[3];
  R=y[4];
#
# ODEs
  St=(1-eps)+omega*V+delta*R-beta*S*I-xi*S-S;
  Vt=xi*S-(1-sigma)*beta*V*I-(1+omega)*V;
  It=eps+beta*S*I+(1-sigma)*beta*V*I-
```

```
     (1+alpha)*I;
   Rt=alpha*I-(1+delta)*R;
#
# Four scalars to one vector
   yt=rep(0,4);
   yt[1]=St;
   yt[2]=Vt;
   yt[3]=It;
   yt[4]=Rt;
#
# Increment calls to ode1a
   ncall <<- ncall+1;
#
# Return derivative vector
   return(list(c(yt)));
   }
```

Listing 4.2: ODE routine for eqs. (3.3)

We can note the following details about **ode1a**.

- The function is defined.

  ```
  ode1a=function(t,y,parm){
  #
  # Function pde1a computes the t derivatives
  # of S(t),V(t),I(t),R(t)
  ```

  t is the current value of t in eqs. (3.3). y is the 4-vector of ODE dependent variables. **parm** is an argument to pass parameters to **ode1a** (unused, but required in the argument list). The arguments must be listed in the order stated to properly interface with **lsodes** called in the main program of Listing 4.1. The derivative vector of the LHS of eqs. (3.3) is calculated and returned to **lsodes** as explained subsequently.

- Vector **y** is placed in four scalars to facilitate the programming of eqs. (3.3).

```
#
# One vector to four scalars
  S=y[1];
  V=y[2];
  I=y[3];
  R=y[4];
```

- Eqs. (3.3) are coded.

```
#
# ODEs
  St=(1-eps)+omega*V+delta*R-beta*S*I-xi*S-S;
  Vt=xi*S-(1-sigma)*beta*V*I-(1+omega)*V;
  It=eps+beta*S*I+(1-sigma)*beta*V*I-
     (1+alpha)*I;
  Rt=alpha*I-(1+delta)*R;
```

For example, eq. (3.3-1) is programmed as

```
  St=(1-eps)+omega*V+delta*R-beta*S*I-xi*S-S;
```

to give the derivative $\dfrac{dS(t)}{dt} = $ St.

- The four scalar derivatives $\dfrac{dS(t)}{dt} = $ St, $\dfrac{dV(t)}{dt} = $ Vt, $\dfrac{dI(t)}{dt} = $ It, $\dfrac{dR(t)}{dt} = $ Rt are placed in a vector **yt** to return to **lsodes** for the next step along the solution.

```
#
# Four scalars to one vector
  yt=rep(0,4);
  yt[1]=St;
  yt[2]=Vt;
  yt[3]=It;
  yt[4]=Rt;
```

- The number of calls to odela is incremented and returned to the main program of Listing 4.1 with <<-.

```
#
# Increment calls to odela
   ncall <<- ncall+1;
```

- The derivative vector yt is returned to lsodes as a list as required by lsodes.

```
#
# Return derivative vector
   return(list(c(yt)));
   }
```

c is the R numerical vector operator. The final } terminates function odela.

This completes the discussion of odela. The numerical and graphical output from the R routines of Listings 4.1, 4.2 is considered next.

(4.1.3) Numerical and graphical output

The numerical output for from the R routines of Listings 4.1, 4.2 follows.

```
[1] 21

[1] 5


t =     0.00  S =    1.000
t =     0.00  V =    0.000
t =     0.00  I =    0.000
t =     0.00  R =    0.000

t =     0.50  S =    0.125
t =     0.50  V =    0.648
```

```
t =      0.50   I =   0.219
t =      0.50   R =   0.009

t =      1.00   S =   0.090
t =      1.00   V =   0.356
t =      1.00   I =   0.519
t =      1.00   R =   0.035

t =      1.50   S =   0.074
t =      1.50   V =   0.204
t =      1.50   I =   0.661
t =      1.50   R =   0.062

t =      2.00   S =   0.070
t =      2.00   V =   0.164
t =      2.00   I =   0.689
t =      2.00   R =   0.077

ncall =     120
```

Table 4.1: Numerical output from Listings 4.1, 4.2

We can note the following details about this output.

- 21 t output points as the first dimension of the solution matrix out from lsodes as programmed in the main program of Listing 4.1 (with nout=21).
- The solution matrix out returned by lsodes has 5 elements as a second dimension. The first element is the value of t. Elements 2 to 5 are $S(t), V(t), I(t), R(t)$.
- The solution is displayed for t=0,2/20,...,2 as programmed in Listing 4.1 (every fifth value of t is displayed as explained previously).
- ICs (3.5) are confirmed, $S(t=0) = 1, V(t=0) = I(t=0) = R(t=0) = 0$.

- The solutions appear to be approaching a stable steady state, which is confirmed in the graphical output of Fig. 4.1.
- `lsodes` computes the solution to the 4×4 ODE system efficiently, `ncall=120`.

Fig. 4.1 indicates a gridding effect (nonsmooth solution in t), which suggests a larger value of `nout`. This is left as an exercise.

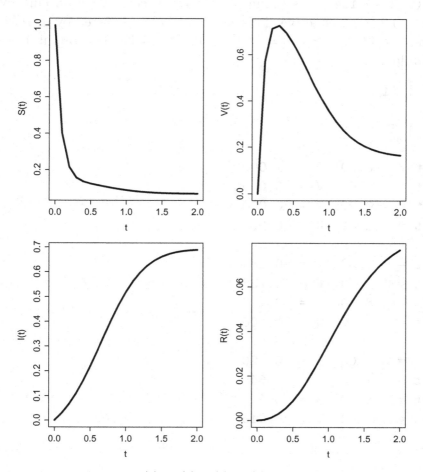

Figure 4.1: $S(t), V(t), I(t), R(t)$ from eqs. (3.3)

The final output in Table 4.1,

```
t =     2.00  S =   0.070
t =     2.00  V =   0.164
t =     2.00  I =   0.689
t =     2.00  R =   0.077
```

indicates a relatively large value of the infected population, $I(t=2) = 0.689$, and a small vaccinated population, $V(t=2)=0.164$. This suggests that the vaccine with an efficacy $\sigma = 0.2$ is not effective. This conclusion can be tested by increasing the efficacy to $\sigma = 0.9$ (in Listing 4.1). The ouput is in Table 4.2.

[1] 21

[1] 5


```
t =     0.00  S =   1.000
t =     0.00  V =   0.000
t =     0.00  I =   0.000
t =     0.00  R =   0.000

t =     0.50  S =   0.134
t =     0.50  V =   0.738
t =     0.50  I =   0.122
t =     0.50  R =   0.006

t =     1.00  S =   0.120
t =     1.00  V =   0.649
t =     1.00  I =   0.215
t =     1.00  R =   0.016
```

```
t =      1.50   S =    0.112
t =      1.50   V =    0.579
t =      1.50   I =    0.283
t =      1.50   R =    0.026

t =      2.00   S =    0.106
t =      2.00   V =    0.531
t =      2.00   I =    0.329
t =      2.00   R =    0.034

ncall =      114
```

Table 4.2: Numerical output from Listings 4.1, 4.2, $\sigma = 0.9$

The graphical output is in Fig. 4.2.

```
sigma=0.2

t =      2.00   S =    0.070
t =      2.00   V =    0.164
t =      2.00   I =    0.689
t =      2.00   R =    0.077

sigma=0.9

t =      2.00   S =    0.106
t =      2.00   V =    0.531
t =      2.00   I =    0.329
t =      2.00   R =    0.034
```

The substantial reduction in the infected population, $I(t)$, and increase in the vaccinated population, $V(t)$, resulting from the increase in the vaccine efficacy is clear.

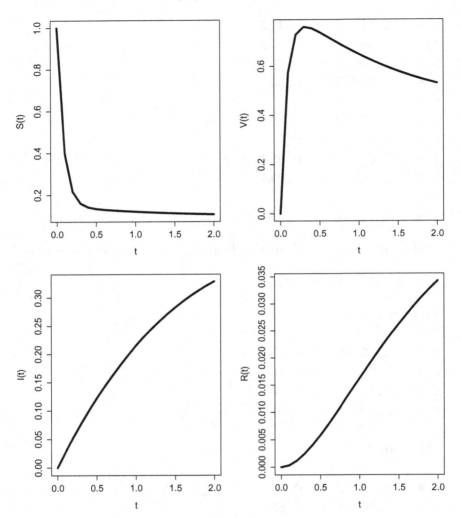

Figure 4.2: $S(t), V(t), I(t), R(t)$ from eqs. (3.3), $\sigma = 0.9$

The solution properties in Figs. 4.1, 4.2 are determined by the derivatives $\dfrac{dS(t)}{dt}$, $\dfrac{dV(t)}{dt}$, $\dfrac{dI(t)}{dt}$, $\dfrac{dR(t)}{dt}$ defined by eqs. (3.3), These derivatives are computed and displayed with the following code added to Listing 4.1.

```
#
# Plot ODE derivatives
#
# dS/dt
  par(mfrow=c(2,2));
  St=rep(0,nout);
  for(it in 1:nout){
    St[it]=(1-eps)+omega*V[it]+delta*R[it]-
           beta*S[it]*I[it]-xi*S[it]-S[it];}
  matplot(x=t,y=St,type="l",xlab="t",ylab="dS(t)/dt",
    xlim=c(t0,tf),lty=1,main="",lwd=2,col="black");
#
# dV/dt
  Vt=rep(0,nout);
  for(it in 1:nout){
    Vt[it]=xi*S[it]-(1-sigma)*beta*V[it]*I[it]-
           (1+omega)*V[it];}
  matplot(x=t,y=Vt,type="l",xlab="t",ylab="dV(t)/dt",
    xlim=c(t0,tf),lty=1,main="",lwd=2,col="black");
#
# dI/dt
  It=rep(0,nout);
  for(it in 1:nout){
    It[it]=eps+beta*S[it]*I[it]+(1-sigma)*
```

```
            beta*V[it]*I[it]-(1+alpha)*I[it];}
     matplot(x=t,y=It,type="l",xlab="t",ylab="dI(t)/dt",
       xlim=c(t0,tf),lty=1,main="",lwd=2,col="black");
#
# dR/dt
  Rt=rep(0,nout);
  for(it in 1:nout){
    Rt[it]=alpha*I[it]-(1+delta)*R[it];}
  matplot(x=t,y=Rt,type="l",xlab="t",ylab="dR(t)/dt",
    xlim=c(t0,tf),lty=1,main="",lwd=2,col="black");
```

Listing 4.3: Code added to Listing 4.1 to compute and display
the derivatives of eqs. (3.3)

The programming of the calculation of the derivatives in t is
taken from **ode1a**, with the addition of a subscript for t. For
example, for $\dfrac{dS(t)}{dt}$, the programing from **ode1a**,

```
St=(1-eps)+omega*V+delta*R-beta*S*I-xi*S-S;
```

is modified to

```
St[it]=(1-eps)+omega*V[it]+delta*R[it]-
beta*S[it]*I[it]-xi*S[it]-S[it];
```

through the addition of the subscript **it** in Listing 4.3.

The graphical output is in Fig. 4.3

Fig. 4.3 indicates the approach to a steady state as the
derivatives in t approach zero. The largest derivatives are at
$t = 0$, which is typically the case for dynamic models.

To gain further insight into the properties of the derivatives,
the RHS terms of eqs. (3.3) can be computed and displayed.

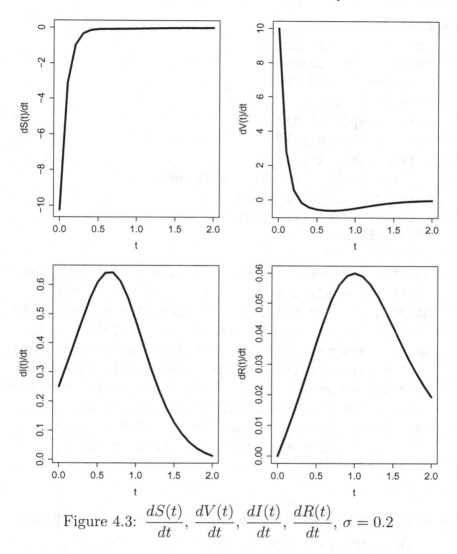

Figure 4.3: $\dfrac{dS(t)}{dt}$, $\dfrac{dV(t)}{dt}$, $\dfrac{dI(t)}{dt}$, $\dfrac{dR(t)}{dt}$, $\sigma = 0.2$

For example, for eq. (3.3-1), the RHS terms are computed and displayed with the following code added to Listing 4.3.

```
#
# Plot ODE RHS terms
#
```

```
# S(t)
  term11=rep(0,nout);
  term12=rep(0,nout);
  term13=rep(0,nout);
  term14=rep(0,nout);
  term15=rep(0,nout);
  for (it in 1:nout){
    term11[it]=1-eps;
    term12[it]=omega*V[it]+delta*R[it];
    term13[it]=-beta*S[it]*I[it];
    term14[it]=-(1+xi)*S[it];
    term15[it]=St[it];}
  par(mfrow=c(3,2));
  matplot(x=t,y=term11,type="l",xlab="t",ylab="term11",
    xlim=c(t0,tf),lty=1,main="",lwd=2,col="black");
  matplot(x=t,y=term12,type="l",xlab="t",ylab="term12",
    xlim=c(t0,tf),lty=1,main="",lwd=2,col="black");
  matplot(x=t,y=term13,type="l",xlab="t",ylab="term13",
    xlim=c(t0,tf),lty=1,main="",lwd=2,col="black");
  matplot(x=t,y=term14,type="l",xlab="t",ylab="term14",
    xlim=c(t0,tf),lty=1,main="",lwd=2,col="black");
  matplot(x=t,y=term15,type="l",xlab="t",ylab="term15=
    dS(t)/dt",xlim=c(t0,tf),lty=1,main="",lwd=2,
    col="black");
```

Listing 4.4: Code added to Listing 4.3 to compute and display the RHS terms of the derivative $\dfrac{dS(t)}{dt}$ of eq. (3.3-1).

The notation for the terms is **term1n** where the 1 refers to eq. (3.3-1) and n refers to the number of the RHS term in eq. (3.3-1) with n=1,2,3,4,5.

The graphical output from Listing 4.4 follows.

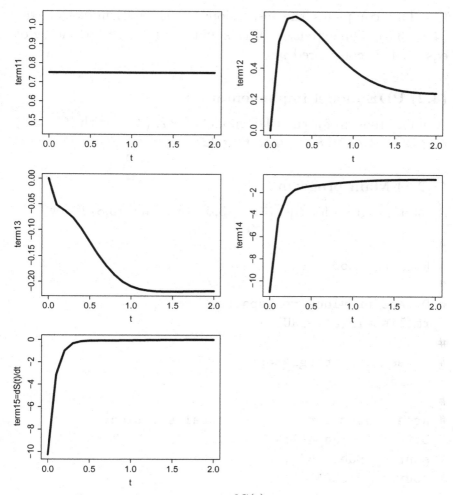

Figure 4.4: RHS terms of $\dfrac{dS(t)}{dt}$, eq. (3.3-1), $\sigma = 0.2$

Fig. 4.4 indicates `term14[it]=-(1+xi)*S[it]` is the largest contributor to the derivative $\dfrac{dS(t)}{dt}$, principally from the value of $\xi = $ `xi=10`. `term15` $= \dfrac{dS(t)}{dt}$ of Fig. 4.3.

This completes the discussion of the ODE model of eqs. (3.3) (3.5), The extension of this analysis to the PDE model of eqs. (3.4) is considered next.

(4.2) PDE model implementation

A main program for the PDE model of eqs. (3.4), with ICs (3.6) and BCs (3.7), (3.8) is in Listing 4.5.

(4.2.1) Main program

A main program for eqs. (3.4), (3.6), (3.7) and (3.8) follows

```
#
# Four PDE model
#
# Delete previous workspaces
  rm(list=ls(all=TRUE))
#
# Access ODE integrator
  library("deSolve");
#
# Access functions for numerical solution
  setwd("f:/chap4");
  source("pde1a.R");
  source("dss004.R");
#
# Parameters
  alpha=0.25;
  beta=4.5;
  delta=1;
  eps=0.25;
  xi=10;
  omega=1;
  sigma=0.2;
```

```
  Ds=1.0e-00; Dv=1.0e-00;
  Di=1.0e-00; Dr=1.0e-00;
  ks=0; kv=0; ki=0; kr=0;
  Sb=1; Vb=1; Ib=1; Rb=1;
#
# Spatial grid (in r)
  nr=21;rl=0;ru=1;dr=(ru-rl)/(nr-1)
  r=seq(from=rl,to=ru,by=dr);
#
# Independent variable for ODE integration
  t0=0;tf=2;nout=41;
  tout=seq(from=t0,to=tf,by=(tf-t0)/(nout-1));
#
# Initial condition (t=0)
  u0=rep(0,4*nr);
  for(i in 1:nr){
    u0[i]     =1;
    u0[i+nr]  =0;
    u0[i+2*nr]=0;
    u0[i+3*nr]=0;
  }
  ncall=0;
#
# ODE integration
  out=lsodes(y=u0,times=tout,func=pde1a,
      sparsetype ="sparseint",rtol=1e-6,
      atol=1e-6,maxord=5);
  nrow(out)
  ncol(out)
#
# Arrays for plotting numerical solution
  Sp=matrix(0,nrow=nr,ncol=nout);
  Vp=matrix(0,nrow=nr,ncol=nout);
  Ip=matrix(0,nrow=nr,ncol=nout);
```

```
Rp=matrix(0,nrow=nr,ncol=nout);
for(it in 1:nout){
  for(i in 1:nr){
    Sp[i,it]=out[it,i+1];
    Vp[i,it]=out[it,i+1+nr];
    Ip[i,it]=out[it,i+1+2*nr];
    Rp[i,it]=out[it,i+1+3*nr];
  }
}
#
# Display numerical solution
  iv=seq(from=1,to=nout,by=20);
  for(it in iv){
    cat(sprintf("\n     t      r       S(r,t)
                \n"));
    iv=seq(from=1,to=nr,by=10);
    for(i in iv){
      cat(sprintf("%6.2f%6.2f%10.3f\n",
          tout[it],r[i],Sp[i,it]));
    }
    cat(sprintf("\n     t      r       V(r,t)
                \n"));
    iv=seq(from=1,to=nr,by=10);
    for(i in iv){
      cat(sprintf("%6.2f%6.2f%10.3f\n",
          tout[it],r[i],Vp[i,it]));
    }
    cat(sprintf("\n     t      r       I(r,t)
                \n"));
    iv=seq(from=1,to=nr,by=10);
    for(i in iv){
      cat(sprintf("%6.2f%6.2f%10.3f\n",
          tout[it],r[i],Ip[i,it]));
    }
```

```
    cat(sprintf("\n    t     r       R(r,t)
                \n"));
    iv=seq(from=1,to=nr,by=10);
    for(i in iv){
      cat(sprintf("%6.2f%6.2f%10.3f\n",
          tout[it],r[i],Rp[i,it]));
      }
  }
#
# Calls to ODE routine
  cat(sprintf("\n\n ncall = %5d\n\n",ncall));
#
# Plot PDE solutions
#
# 2D
#
# S(r,t)
  par(mfrow=c(2,2));
  matplot(x=r,y=Sp,type="l",xlab="r",
    ylab="S(r,t)",xlim=c(rl,ru),lty=1,
    main="",lwd=2,col="black");
#
# V(r,t)
  matplot(x=r,y=Vp,type="l",xlab="r",
    ylab="V(r,t)",xlim=c(rl,ru),lty=1,
    main="",lwd=2,col="black");
#
# I(r,t)
  matplot(x=r,y=Ip,type="l",xlab="r",
    ylab="I(r,t)",xlim=c(rl,ru),lty=1,
    main="",lwd=2,col="black");
#
# R(r,t)
  matplot(x=r,y=Rp,type="l",xlab="r",
```

```
    ylab="R(r,t)",xlim=c(rl,ru),lty=1,
    main="",lwd=2,col="black");
#
# 3D
#
# S(r,t)
  par(mfrow=c(2,2));
  persp(r,tout,Sp,theta=45,phi=30,
        xlim=c(rl,ru),ylim=c(t0,tf),xlab="r",
        ylab="t",zlab="S(r,t)");
#
# V(r,t)
  persp(r,tout,Vp,theta=60,phi=30,
        xlim=c(rl,ru),ylim=c(t0,tf),xlab="r",
        ylab="t",zlab="V(r,t)");
#
# I(r,t)
  persp(r,tout,Ip,theta=60,phi=30,
        xlim=c(rl,ru),ylim=c(t0,tf),xlab="r",
        ylab="t",zlab="I(r,t)");
#
# R(r,t)
  persp(r,tout,Rp,theta=60,phi=30,
        xlim=c(rl,ru),ylim=c(t0,tf),xlab="r",
        ylab="t",zlab="R(r,t)");
```

Listing 4.5: Main program for eqs. (3.4), (3.6), (3.7), (3.8)

We can note the following details about Listing 4.5 (with some repetition of the discussion of Listing 4.1 so that the following discussion is self contained).

- Previous workspaces are deleted.

```
#
#  Four PDE model
#
# Delete previous workspaces
  rm(list=ls(all=TRUE))
```

- The R ODE integrator library `deSolve` is accessed [2]. Then the directory with the files for the solution of eqs. (3.4) is designated. Note that `setwd` (set working directory) uses / rather than the usual \.

```
#
# Access ODE integrator
  library("deSolve");
#
# Access functions for numerical solution
  setwd("f:/chap4");
  source("pde1a.R");
  source("dss004.R");
```

`pde1a` is the ODE method of lines (MOL) routine for eqs. (3.4), (3.6), (3.7), (3.8), discussed subsequently. `dss004` is a library routine for calculating spatial first derivatives (called in `pde1a` and listed in Appendix A).

- The model parameters are specified numerically.

```
#
# Parameters
  alpha=0.25;
  beta=4.5;
  delta=1;
  eps=0.25;
```

```
xi=10;
omega=1;
sigma=0.2;
Ds=1.0e-00; Dv=1.0e-00;
Di=1.0e-00; Dr=1.0e-00;
ks=0; kv=0; ki=0; kr=0;
Sb=1; Vb=1; Ib=1; Rb=1;
```

We can note the following details about these parameters.

- Parameters `alpha` to `sigma` are the same as in Listing 4.1. In particular, the vaccine efficacy is `sigma=0.2`.
- The diffusivities `Ds`, `Dv`, `Di`, `Dr` are defined numerically.
- The transfer coefficients `ks`, `kv`, `ki`, `kr` are zero so that eqs. (3.8) are homogeneous (zero) Neumann (no flux) BCs.
- The ambient population densities, `Sb`, `Sv`, `Si`, `Sb` are nonzeo.

This combination of parameters provides a test of the coding of the PDE model as explained subsequently.

- A spatial grid for eqs. (3.4) is defined with 21 points so that $r = 0, 0.05, \ldots, 1$.

```
#
# Spatial grid (in r)
  nr=21;rl=0;ru=1;dr=(ru-rl)/(nr-1)
  r=seq(from=rl,to=ru,by=dr);
```

- An interval in t is defined for 41 output points, so that $\text{tout}=0, 2/40, \ldots, 2$ (yr).

```
#
# Independent variable for ODE integration
  t0=0;tf=2;nout=41;
  tout=seq(from=t0,to=tf,by=(tf-t0)/(nout-1));
```

With `nout=21`, the `lsodes` integration in t develops an instability. The increase to `nout=41` eliminates the instability (the PDE solutions from eqs. (3.4) proceed to a stable steady state as reflected in the subsequent Table 4.3).

- ICs (3.6) are implemented. $S(r, t = 0) = 1$ is placed in a vector u0, followed by $V(r, t = 0) = I(r, t = 0) = R(r, t = 0) = 0$.

```
#
# Initial condition (t=0)
  u0=rep(0,4*nr);
  for(i in 1:nr){
    u0[i]     =1;
    u0[i+nr]  =0;
    u0[i+2*nr]=0;
    u0[i+3*nr]=0;
  }
  ncall=0;
```

Also, the counter for the calls to `pde1a` is initialized.

- The system of (4)21 = 84 ODEs is integrated by the library integrator `lsodes` (available in `deSolve`, [2]). As expected, the inputs to `lsodes` are the ODE function, `pde1a`, the IC vector u0, and the vector of output values of t, `tout`. The length of u0 (84) informs `lsodes` how many ODEs are to be integrated. `func,y,times` are reserved names.

```
#
# ODE integration
  out=lsodes(y=u0,times=tout,func=pde1a,
      sparsetype ="sparseint",rtol=1e-6,
      atol=1e-6,maxord=5);
  nrow(out)
  ncol(out)
```

`nrow,ncol` confirm the dimensions of `out`.

- $S(r, t), V(r, t), I(r, t), R(r, t)$ are placed in matrices for subsequent plotting.

```
#
# Arrays for plotting numerical solution
  Sp=matrix(0,nrow=nr,ncol=nout);
  Vp=matrix(0,nrow=nr,ncol=nout);
  Ip=matrix(0,nrow=nr,ncol=nout);
  Rp=matrix(0,nrow=nr,ncol=nout);
  for(it in 1:nout){
    for(i in 1:nr){
      Sp[i,it]=out[it,i+1];
      Vp[i,it]=out[it,i+1+nr];
      Ip[i,it]=out[it,i+1+2*nr];
      Rp[i,it]=out[it,i+1+3*nr];
    }
  }
```

The offset +1 is required since the first element of the solution vectors in out is the value of t and the 2 to 85 elements are the 4(41) values of $S(r, t), V(r, t), I(r, t), R(r, t)$. These dimensions from the preceding calls to nrow,ncol are confirmed in the subsequent output.

- $S(r, t), V(r, t), I(r, t), R(r, t)$ are displayed as a function of r, t with two fors. Every 20th value of t is displayed with by=20 and every 10th value of r is displayed with by=10.

```
#
# Display numerical solution
  iv=seq(from=1,to=nout,by=20);
  for(it in iv){
    cat(sprintf("\n    t      r       S(r,t)
                 \n"));
```

```
    iv=seq(from=1,to=nr,by=10);
    for(i in iv){
      cat(sprintf("%6.1f%6.1f%12.3e\n",
          tout[it],r[i],Sp[i,it]));
    }
    cat(sprintf("\n      t      r       V(r,t)
                  \n"));
    iv=seq(from=1,to=nr,by=10);
    for(i in iv){
      cat(sprintf("%6.1f%6.1f%12.3e\n",
          tout[it],r[i],Vp[i,it]));
    }
    cat(sprintf("\n      t      r       I(r,t)
                  \n"));
    iv=seq(from=1,to=nr,by=10);
    for(i in iv){
      cat(sprintf("%6.1f%6.1f%12.3e\n",
          tout[it],r[i],Ip[i,it]));
    }
    cat(sprintf("\n      t      r       R(r,t)
                  \n"));
    iv=seq(from=1,to=nr,by=10);
    for(i in iv){
      cat(sprintf("%6.1f%6.1f%12.3e\n",
          tout[it],r[i],Rp[i,it]));
    }
  }
```

- The number of calls to pde1a is displayed at the end of the solution.

```
#
# Calls to ODE routine
  cat(sprintf("\n\n ncall = %5d\n\n",ncall));
```

- $S(r,t), V(r,t), I(r,t), R(r,t)$ are plotted as a function of r, t in 2D with `matplot` and in 3D with `persp`.

```
#
# Plot PDE solutions
#
# 2D
#
# S(r,t)
  par(mfrow=c(2,2));
  matplot(x=r,y=Sp,type="l",xlab="r",
    ylab="S(r,t)",xlim=c(rl,ru),lty=1,
    main="",lwd=2,col="black");
#
# V(r,t)
  matplot(x=r,y=Vp,type="l",xlab="r",
    ylab="V(r,t)",xlim=c(rl,ru),lty=1,
    main="",lwd=2,col="black");

#
# I(r,t)
  matplot(x=r,y=Ip,type="l",xlab="r",
    ylab="I(r,t)",xlim=c(rl,ru),lty=1,
    main="",lwd=2,col="black");
#
# R(r,t)
  matplot(x=r,y=Rp,type="l",xlab="r",
    ylab="R(r,t)",xlim=c(rl,ru),lty=1,
    main="",lwd=2,col="black");
#
# 3D
#
# S(r,t)
  par(mfrow=c(2,2));
```

```
      persp(r,tout,Sp,theta=45,phi=30,
            xlim=c(rl,ru),ylim=c(t0,tf),xlab="r",
            ylab="t",zlab="S(r,t)");
#
# V(r,t)
      persp(r,tout,Vp,theta=60,phi=30,
            xlim=c(rl,ru),ylim=c(t0,tf),xlab="r",
            ylab="t",zlab="V(r,t)");
#
# I(r,t)
      persp(r,tout,Ip,theta=60,phi=30,
            xlim=c(rl,ru),ylim=c(t0,tf),xlab="r",
            ylab="t",zlab="I(r,t)");
#
# R(r,t)
      persp(r,tout,Rp,theta=60,phi=30,
            xlim=c(rl,ru),ylim=c(t0,tf),xlab="r",
            ylab="t",zlab="R(r,t)");
```

This completes the discussion of the main program in Listing 4.5. The ODE/MOL routine called by `lsodes` in the main program is considered next.

(4.2.2) ODE/MOL routine

The ODE/MOL routine for eqs. (3.4), (3.7), (3.8) follows.

```
  pde1a=function(t,u,parm){
#
# Function pde1a computes the t derivatives
# of S(r,t),V(r,t),I(r,t),R(r,t)
#
# One vector to four vectors
  S=rep(0,nr);
  V=rep(0,nr);
  I=rep(0,nr);
```

```
  R=rep(0,nr);
  for(i in 1:nr){
    S[i]=u[i];
    V[i]=u[i+nr];
    I[i]=u[i+2*nr];
    R[i]=u[i+3*nr];}
#
# First derivatives Sr,Vr,Ir,Rr
  Sr=dss004(rl,ru,nr,S);
  Vr=dss004(rl,ru,nr,V);
  Ir=dss004(rl,ru,nr,I);
  Rr=dss004(rl,ru,nr,R);
#
# BCs
  Sr[1]=0;
  Vr[1]=0;
  Ir[1]=0;
  Rr[1]=0;
  Sr[nr]=(1/Ds)*ks*(Sb-S[nr]));
  Vr[nr]=(1/Dv)*kv*(Vb-V[nr]));
  Ir[nr]=(1/Di)*ki*(Ib-I[nr]));
  Rr[nr]=(1/Dr)*kr*(Rb-R[nr]));
#
# Product functions
  SI=rep(0,nr);
  VI=rep(0,nr);
  for(i in 1:nr){
    SI[i]=S[i]*I[i];
    VI[i]=V[i]*I[i];}
#
# Second derivatives
  Srr=dss004(rl,ru,nr,Sr);
  Vrr=dss004(rl,ru,nr,Vr);
  Irr=dss004(rl,ru,nr,Ir);
```

```
  Rrr=dss004(rl,ru,nr,Rr);
#
# PDEs
  St=rep(0,nr);
  Vt=rep(0,nr);
  It=rep(0,nr);
  Rt=rep(0,nr);
  for(i in 1:nr){
    if(i==1){
      St[i]=Ds*2*Srr[i]+
            (1-eps)+omega*V[i]+delta*R[i]-
            beta*SI[i]-xi*S[i]-S[i];
      Vt[i]=Dv*2*Vrr[i]+
            xi*S[i]-(1-sigma)*beta*VI[i]-
            (1+omega)*V[i];
      It[i]=Di*2*Irr[i]+
            eps+beta*SI[i]+(1-sigma)*beta*VI[i]-
            (1+alpha)*I[i];
      Rt[i]=Dr*2*Rrr[i]+
            alpha*I[i]-(1+delta)*R[i];
    }
    if(i>1){
      St[i]=Ds*(Srr[i]+(1/r[i])*Sr[i])+
            (1-eps)+omega*V[i]+delta*R[i]-
            beta*SI[i]-xi*S[i]-S[i];
      Vt[i]=Dv*(Vrr[i]+(1/r[i])*Vr[i])+
            xi*S[i]-(1-sigma)*beta*VI[i]-
            (1+omega)*V[i];
      It[i]=Di*(Irr[i]+(1/r[i])*Ir[i])+
            eps+beta*SI[i]+(1-sigma)*beta*VI[i]-
            (1+alpha)*I[i];
      Rt[i]=Dr*(Rrr[i]+(1/r[i])*Rr[i])+
            alpha*I[i]-(1+delta)*R[i];
    }
```

```
#
# Next r
  }
#
# Four vectors to one vector
  ut=rep(0,4*nr);
  for(i in 1:nr){
    ut[i]     =St[i];
    ut[i+nr]   =Vt[i];
    ut[i+2*nr]=It[i];
    ut[i+3*nr]=Rt[i];
  }
#
# Increment calls to pde1a
  ncall <<- ncall+1;
#
# Return derivative vector
  return(list(c(ut)));
  }
```

Listing 4.6: ODE/MOL routine `pde1a` for eqs. (3.4), (3.7), (3.8)

We can note the following details about Listing 4.6.

- The function is defined.

```
pde1a=function(t,u,parm){
#
# Function pde1a computes the t derivatives
# of S(r,t),V(r,t),I(r,t),R(r,t)
```

t is the current value of t in eqs. (3.4). u is the 84-vector of ODE/MOL dependent variables. parm is an argument to pass parameters to pde1a (unused, but required in the argument list). The arguments must be listed in the order stated to properly interface with lsodes called in the main program of Listing 4.5. The LHS t derivative vectors of eqs. (3.4) are calculated and returned to lsodes as explained subsequently.

- Vector u is placed in four vectors to facilitate the programming of the MOL integration (solution) of eqs. (3.4), (3.7), (3.8) [1].

```
#
# One vector to four vectors
  S=rep(0,nr);
  V=rep(0,nr);
  I=rep(0,nr);
  R=rep(0,nr);
  for(i in 1:nr){
    S[i]=u[i];
    V[i]=u[i+nr];
    I[i]=u[i+2*nr];
    R[i]=u[i+3*nr];}
```

- $\dfrac{\partial S(r,t)}{\partial r}, \dfrac{\partial V(r,t)}{\partial r}, \dfrac{\partial I(r,t)}{\partial r}, \dfrac{\partial R(r,t)}{\partial r}$ are computed.

```
#
# First derivatives Sr,Vr,Ir,Rr
  Sr=dss004(rl,ru,nr,S);
  Vr=dss004(rl,ru,nr,V);
  Ir=dss004(rl,ru,nr,I);
  Rr=dss004(rl,ru,nr,R);
```

- BCs (3.7) are programmed. Subscript 1 pertains to $r = r_l = 0$.

```
#
# BCs
  Sr[1]=0;
  Vr[1]=0;
```

```
Ir[1]=0;
Rr[1]=0;
```

- BCs (3.8) are programmed. Subscript `nr` pertains to $r = r_u = 1$.

```
Sr[nr]=(1/Ds)*ks*(Sb-S[nr]);
Vr[nr]=(1/Dv)*kv*(Vb-V[nr]);
Ir[nr]=(1/Di)*ki*(Ib-I[nr]);
Rr[nr]=(1/Dr)*kr*(Rb-R[nr]);
```

- The product functions $S(r,t)I(r,t)$, $V(r,t)I(r,t)$ are computed.

```
#
# Product functions
  SI=rep(0,nr);
  VI=rep(0,nr);
  for(i in 1:nr){
    SI[i]=S[i]*I[i];
    VI[i]=V[i]*I[i];}
```

- $\dfrac{\partial^2 S(r,t)}{\partial r^2}$, $\dfrac{\partial^2 V(r,t)}{\partial r^2}$, $\dfrac{\partial^2 I(r,t)}{\partial r^2}$, $\dfrac{\partial^2 R(r,t)}{\partial r^2}$, are computed.

```
#
# Second derivatives
  Srr=dss004(rl,ru,nr,Sr);
  Vrr=dss004(rl,ru,nr,Vr);
  Irr=dss004(rl,ru,nr,Ir);
  Rrr=dss004(rl,ru,nr,Rr);
```

- PDEs (3.4) are programmed for $r = r_l = 0$.

```
#
# PDEs
  St=rep(0,nr);
  Vt=rep(0,nr);
```

```
It=rep(0,nr);
Rt=rep(0,nr);
for(i in 1:nr){
  if(i==1){
    St[i]=Ds*2*Srr[i]+
          (1-eps)+omega*V[i]+delta*R[i]-
          beta*SI[i]-xi*S[i]-S[i];
    Vt[i]=Dv*2*Vrr[i]+
          xi*S[i]-(1-sigma)*beta*VI[i]-
          (1+omega)*V[i];
    It[i]=Di*2*Irr[i]+
          eps+beta*SI[i]+(1-sigma)*beta*VI[i]-
          (1+alpha)*I[i];
    Rt[i]=Dr*2*Rrr[i]+
          alpha*I[i]-(1+delta)*R[i];
  }
```

The singularities of the radial groups at $r = 0$, $\dfrac{1}{r}\dfrac{\partial S(r,t)}{\partial r}$, $\dfrac{1}{r}\dfrac{\partial V(r,t)}{\partial r}$, $\dfrac{1}{r}\dfrac{\partial I(r,t)}{\partial r}$, $\dfrac{1}{r}\dfrac{\partial R(r,t)}{\partial r}$, are resolved by l'Hospital's rule. For example, for the self diffusion of $S(r,t)$ (with the use of BC (3.7-1)),

$$\frac{1}{r}\left(\frac{\partial S(r,t)}{\partial r}\right)\Big|_{r\to 0} = \frac{\partial^2 S(r,t)}{\partial r^2}$$

- PDEs (3.4) are programmed for $r > 0$.

```
    if(i>1){
      St[i]=Ds*(Srr[i]+(1/r[i])*Sr[i])+
            (1-eps)+omega*V[i]+delta*R[i]-
            beta*SI[i]-xi*S[i]-S[i];
      Vt[i]=Dv*(Vrr[i]+(1/r[i])*Vr[i])+
            xi*S[i]-(1-sigma)*beta*VI[i]-
            (1+omega)*V[i];
```

```
It[i]=Di*(Irr[i]+(1/r[i])*Ir[i])+
      eps+beta*SI[i]+(1-sigma)*beta*VI[i]-
      (1+alpha)*I[i];
Rt[i]=Dr*(Rrr[i]+(1/r[i])*Rr[i])+
      alpha*I[i]-(1+delta)*R[i];
}
```

The `for` is concluded for stepping through the values of r.

```
#
# Next r
}
```

- The four derivatives in t of eqs. (3.4), $\dfrac{\partial S(r,t)}{\partial t}$, $\dfrac{\partial V(r,t)}{\partial t}$, $\dfrac{\partial I(r,t)}{\partial t}$, $\dfrac{\partial R(r,t)}{\partial t}$, are placed in a single vector, `ut`, to return to `lsodes` for the next step along the solution.

```
#
# Four vectors to one vector
  ut=rep(0,4*nr);
  for(i in 1:nr){
    ut[i]       =St[i];
    ut[i+nr]    =Vt[i];
    ut[i+2*nr]=It[i];
    ut[i+3*nr]=Rt[i];
  }
```

- The number of calls to `pde1a` is incremented and returned to the main program of Listing 4.5 with `<<-`.

```
#
# Increment calls to pde1a
  ncall <<- ncall+1;
#
```

- The derivative vector ut is returned to lsodes as a list as required by lsodes.

```
#
# Return derivative vector
  return(list(c(ut)));
  }
```

c is the R numerical vector operator. The final } terminates function pde1a.

This completes the discussion of pde1a. The output from the main program and ODE/MOL routine of Listings 4.5, 4.6 is considered next.

(4.2.3) Numerical, graphical output

The numerical output is in Table 4.3.

```
[1] 41

[1] 85
```

t	r	S(r,t)
0.00	0.00	1.000
0.00	0.50	1.000
0.00	1.00	1.000

t	r	V(r,t)
0.00	0.00	0.000
0.00	0.50	0.000
0.00	1.00	0.000

t	r	I(r,t)
0.00	0.00	0.000
0.00	0.50	0.000

0.00	1.00	0.000

t	r	R(r,t)
0.00	0.00	0.000
0.00	0.50	0.000
0.00	1.00	0.000

t	r	S(r,t)
1.00	0.00	0.090
1.00	0.50	0.090
1.00	1.00	0.090

t	r	V(r,t)
1.00	0.00	0.356
1.00	0.50	0.356
1.00	1.00	0.356

t	r	I(r,t)
1.00	0.00	0.519
1.00	0.50	0.519
1.00	1.00	0.519

t	r	R(r,t)
1.00	0.00	0.035
1.00	0.50	0.035
1.00	1.00	0.035

t	r	S(r,t)
2.00	0.00	0.070
2.00	0.50	0.070
2.00	1.00	0.070

t	r	V(r,t)
2.00	0.00	0.164

| 2.00 | 0.50 | 0.164 |
| 2.00 | 1.00 | 0.164 |

t	r	I(r,t)
2.00	0.00	0.689
2.00	0.50	0.689
2.00	1.00	0.689

t	r	R(r,t)
2.00	0.00	0.077
2.00	0.50	0.077
2.00	1.00	0.077

```
ncall =   245
```

Table 4.3: Numerical output from eqs. (3.4), (3.6), (3.7), (3.8)

We can note the following details about this output.

- 41 t output points as the first dimension of the solution matrix out from lsodes as programmed in the main program of Listing 4.5 (with nout=41).
- The solution matrix out returned by lsodes has 85 elements as a second dimension. The first element is the value of t. Elements 2 to 85 are $S(r,t), V(r,t), I(r,t), R(r,t)$.
- The solution is displayed for t=0,2/40,...,2 as programmed in Listing 4.5 (every 20th value of t and every 10th value of r as explained previously).
- ICs (3.6) are confirmed, $S(r, t = 0) = 1$, $V(r, t = 0) = I(r, t = 0) = R(r, t = 0) = 0$.
- The solutions are invariant in r (Table 4.3) since (1) the ICs (3.6) are constant in r and eqs. (3.8) are homogeneous (zero) Neumann (no flux) BCs (from $k_s = k_v = k_i = k_r = 0$) and (2) the spatial derivatives in eqs. (3.4) are

zero (derivatives of constants). This is an important test since any variations of the solutions with r would indicate a modeling/programming error.

- The solutions for the ODE and PDE models are the same, which is a consequence of the invariance in r (so that eqs. (3.4) reduce to eqs. (3.3)).

ODE model, Table 4.1

```
t =    2.00  S =  0.070
t =    2.00  V =  0.164
t =    2.00  I =  0.689
t =    2.00  R =  0.077
```

PDE model, Table 4.3

t	r	S(r,t)
2.00	0.00	0.070
2.00	0.50	0.070
2.00	1.00	0.070

t	r	V(r,t)
2.00	0.00	0.164
2.00	0.50	0.164
2.00	1.00	0.164

t	r	I(r,t)
2.00	0.00	0.689
2.00	0.50	0.689
2.00	1.00	0.689

t	r	R(r,t)
2.00	0.00	0.077
2.00	0.50	0.077
2.00	1.00	0.077

Again, this is an important test since any differences in the ODE/MOL solutions would indicate a modeling/programming error.

- `lsodes` computes the solution to the 4×4 PDE system efficiently, `ncall=245`.

The graphical output is in Figs. 4.5.

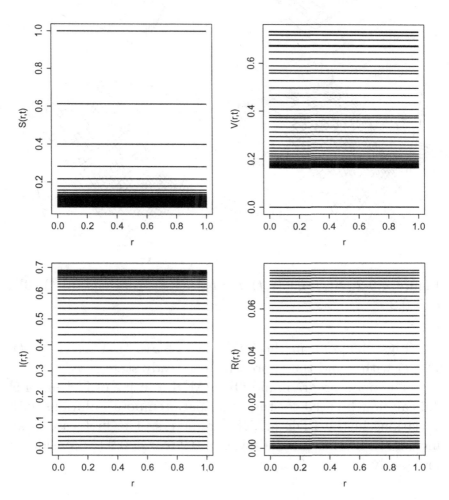

Figure 4.5-1: $S(r,t), V(r,t), I(r,t), R(r,t)$ from eqs. (3.4), 2D, $\sigma = 0.2$

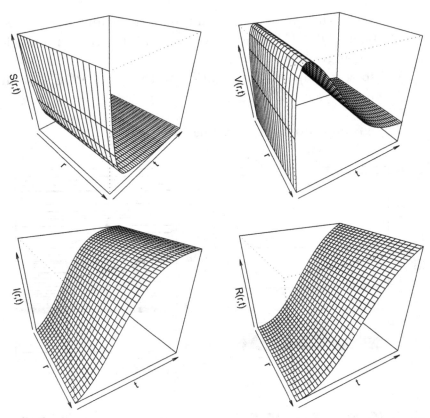

Figure 4.5-2: $S(r,t), V(r,t), I(r,t), R(r,t)$ from eqs. (3.4), 3D, $\sigma = 0.2$

Figs. 4.5 confirm the invariance of $S(r,t)$, $V(r,t)$, $I(r,t)$, $R(r,t)$ with r and the approach to a steady state.

The main program and ODE/MOL routine of Listings 4.5, 4.6 can now be used to study the spatiotemporal solutions with variations in the PDE model parameters. The first case is an increase in the vaccine efficacy, $\sigma = 0.2$ to $\sigma = 0.9$ (as considered previously for eqs. (3.3)).

The numerical output is in Table 4.4.

[1] 41

[1] 85

t	r	S(r,t)
0.00	0.00	1.000
0.00	0.50	1.000
0.00	1.00	1.000

t	r	V(r,t)
0.00	0.00	0.000
0.00	0.50	0.000
0.00	1.00	0.000

t	r	I(r,t)
0.00	0.00	0.000
0.00	0.50	0.000
0.00	1.00	0.000

t	r	R(r,t)
0.00	0.00	0.000
0.00	0.50	0.000
0.00	1.00	0.000

t	r	S(r,t)
1.00	0.00	0.120
1.00	0.50	0.120
1.00	1.00	0.120

t	r	V(r,t)
1.00	0.00	0.649
1.00	0.50	0.649
1.00	1.00	0.649

t	r	I(r,t)
1.00	0.00	0.215
1.00	0.50	0.215
1.00	1.00	0.215

t	r	R(r,t)
1.00	0.00	0.016
1.00	0.50	0.016
1.00	1.00	0.016

t	r	S(r,t)
2.00	0.00	0.106
2.00	0.50	0.106
2.00	1.00	0.106

t	r	V(r,t)
2.00	0.00	0.531
2.00	0.50	0.531
2.00	1.00	0.531

t	r	I(r,t)
2.00	0.00	0.329
2.00	0.50	0.329
2.00	1.00	0.329

t	r	R(r,t)
2.00	0.00	0.034
2.00	0.50	0.034
2.00	1.00	0.034

ncall =   245

Table 4.4: Numerical output from eqs. (3.4), (3.6), (3.7), (3.8), $\sigma = 0.9$

We can note the following details about this output (with some repetition of the previous discussion for $\sigma = 0.2$ after Table 4.3).

- ICs (3.6) are confirmed, $S(r, t = 0) = 1$, $V(r, t = 0) = I(r, t = 0) = R(r, t = 0) = 0$.
- The solutions are invariant in r (Table 4.4) since (1) the ICs (3.6) are constant in r and eqs. (3.8) are homogeneous (zero) Neumann (no flux) BCs (from $k_s = k_v = k_i = k_r = 0$) and (2) the spatial derivatives in eqs. (3.4) are zero (derivatives of constants).
- The solutions for the ODE and PDE models are the same, which is a consequence of the invariance in r (so that eqs. (3.4) reduce to eqs. (3.3)).

```
ODE model, Table 4.2


t =    2.00  S =   0.106
t =    2.00  V =   0.531
t =    2.00  I =   0.329
t =    2.00  R =   0.034


PDE model, Table 4.4


    t      r      S(r,t)
  2.00   0.00     0.106
  2.00   0.50     0.106
  2.00   1.00     0.106


    t      r      V(r,t)
  2.00   0.00     0.531
  2.00   0.50     0.531
  2.00   1.00     0.531
```

t	r	I(r,t)
2.00	0.00	0.329
2.00	0.50	0.329
2.00	1.00	0.329

t	r	R(r,t)
2.00	0.00	0.034
2.00	0.50	0.034
2.00	1.00	0.034

- The increase $\sigma = 0.2$ to $\sigma = 0.9$ increases $V(r,t)$ and reduces $I(r,t)$.

sigma=0.2, Table 4.3

t	r	S(r,t)
2.00	0.00	0.070
2.00	0.50	0.070
2.00	1.00	0.070

t	r	V(r,t)
2.00	0.00	0.164
2.00	0.50	0.164
2.00	1.00	0.164

t	r	I(r,t)
2.00	0.00	0.689
2.00	0.50	0.689
2.00	1.00	0.689

t	r	R(r,t)
2.00	0.00	0.077

```
2.00  0.50       0.077
2.00  1.00       0.077
```

sigma=0.9, Table 4.4

t	r	S(r,t)
2.00	0.00	0.106
2.00	0.50	0.106
2.00	1.00	0.106

t	r	V(r,t)
2.00	0.00	0.531
2.00	0.50	0.531
2.00	1.00	0.531

t	r	I(r,t)
2.00	0.00	0.329
2.00	0.50	0.329
2.00	1.00	0.329

t	r	R(r,t)
2.00	0.00	0.034
2.00	0.50	0.034
2.00	1.00	0.034

- lsodes computes the solution to the 4×4 PDE system efficiently, ncall=245.

The graphical output is in Figs. 4.6.

Figs. 4.6 confirm the invariance of $S(r,t)$, $V(r,t)$, $I(r,t)$, $R(r,t)$ with r and the approach to a steady state.

As the next case, spatial variation of the solutions is included by using ICs (3.6) with variation in r.

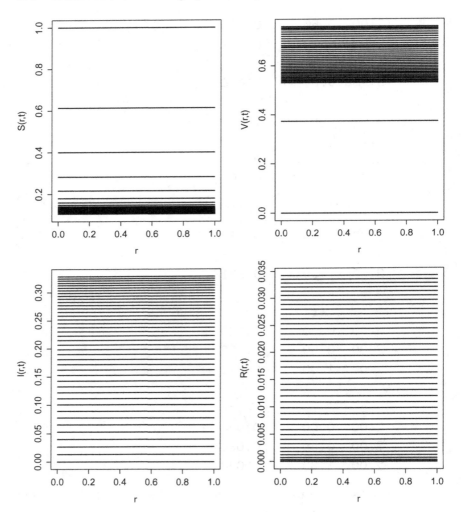

Figure 4.6-1: $S(r,t), V(r,t), I(r,t), R(r,t)$ from eqs. (3.4), 2D, $\sigma = 0.9$

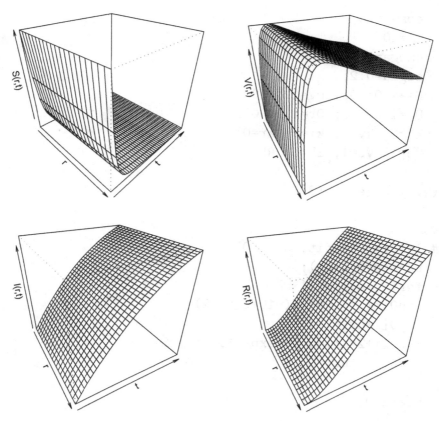

Figure 4.6-2: $S(r,t), V(r,t), I(r,t), R(r,t)$ from eqs. (3.4), 3D, $\sigma = 0.9$

The following changes in the coding in Listing 4.5 were used.

(1) Parameters

```
#
# Parameters
  alpha=0.25;
  beta=4.5;
  delta=1;
```

```
eps=0.25;
xi=10;
omega=1;
sigma=0.2;
Ds=1.0e-03; Dv=1.0e-03;
Di=1.0e-03; Dr=1.0e-03;
ks=0; kv=0; ki=0; kr=0;
Sb=1; Vb=1; Ib=1; Rb=1;
```

(2) ICs (eqs. (3.6))

```
#
# Initial condition (t=0)
  u0=rep(0,4*nr);
  for(i in 1:nr){
     u0[i]      =exp(-10*r[i]^2);
     u0[i+nr]   =0;
     u0[i+2*nr]=0.05*exp(-10*r[i]^2);
     u0[i+3*nr]=0;
  }
  ncall=0;
```

Listing 4.7: Modifications to the main program for eqs. (3.4), (3.6), (3.7), (3.8)

The diffusivities D_S, D_V, D_I, D_R, were selected by trial and error to give smooth variations of the solutions in r. ICs (3.6-1,3) were changed to Gaussian functions centered at $r = 0$, $S(r, t = 0) = e^{-10r^2}$, $I(r, t = 0) = 0.05e^{-10r^2}$. The infected population starts at 5% of the susceptible population.

These Gaussian functions could represent, for example, a large susceptible population in an urban area near $r = 0$

and a smaller susceptible population in an outlying rural area. The model then gives the spatiotemporal dispersion (diffusion, spread) of the four PDE dependent variables with t.

The numerical solution from the main program of Listings 4.5, 4.7 and the ODE/MOL routine **pde1a** of Listing 4.6 follows.

[1] 41

[1] 85

t	r	S(r,t)
0.00	0.00	1.000
0.00	0.50	0.082
0.00	1.00	0.000

t	r	V(r,t)
0.00	0.00	0.000
0.00	0.50	0.000
0.00	1.00	0.000

t	r	I(r,t)
0.00	0.00	0.050
0.00	0.50	0.004
0.00	1.00	0.000

t	r	R(r,t)
0.00	0.00	0.000
0.00	0.50	0.000
0.00	1.00	0.000

t	r	S(r,t)
1.00	0.00	0.082
1.00	0.50	0.088

1.00	1.00	0.087

t	r	$V(r,t)$
1.00	0.00	0.286
1.00	0.50	0.298
1.00	1.00	0.286

t	r	$I(r,t)$
1.00	0.00	0.591
1.00	0.50	0.262
1.00	1.00	0.242

t	r	$R(r,t)$
1.00	0.00	0.045
1.00	0.50	0.018
1.00	1.00	0.017

t	r	$S(r,t)$
2.00	0.00	0.070
2.00	0.50	0.077
2.00	1.00	0.077

t	r	$V(r,t)$
2.00	0.00	0.161
2.00	0.50	0.217
2.00	1.00	0.223

t	r	$I(r,t)$
2.00	0.00	0.686
2.00	0.50	0.533
2.00	1.00	0.515

t	r	$R(r,t)$
2.00	0.00	0.078

```
2.00   0.50        0.051
2.00   1.00        0.049


ncall =    230
```

Table 4.5: Numerical output from eqs. (3.4), (3.6), (3.7), (3.8), $\sigma = 0.2$, $S(r, t = 0) = e^{-10r^2}$, $I(r, t = 0) = 0.05e^{-10r^2}$

We can note the following details about this output (with some repetition of the previous discussion for $\sigma = 0.2$).

- ICs (3.6) are confirmed for $S(r, t = 0) = e^{-10r^2}$, $I(r, t = 0) = 0.05e^{-10r^2}$.
- The vaccinated population increases sharply in t.

```
    t      r      V(r,t)
 0.00   0.00      0.000
 0.00   0.50      0.000
 0.00   1.00      0.000


    t      r      V(r,t)
 2.00   0.00      0.161
 2.00   0.50      0.217
 2.00   1.00      0.223
```

- However, because of the low vaccine efficacy, $\sigma = 0.2$, the infected population also increases sharply in t.

```
    t      r      I(r,t)
 0.00   0.00      0.050
 0.00   0.50      0.004
 0.00   1.00      0.000


    t      r      I(r,t)
 2.00   0.00      0.686
 2.00   0.50      0.533
 2.00   1.00      0.515
```

These features of the solutions are confirmed in Figs. 4.7.

Fig. 4.7-1 indicates the sharp increase in the vaccinated population, $V(r,t)$, but also, the sharp increase in the infected population, $I(r,t)$, resulting from the low vaccine efficacy, $\sigma = 0.2$.

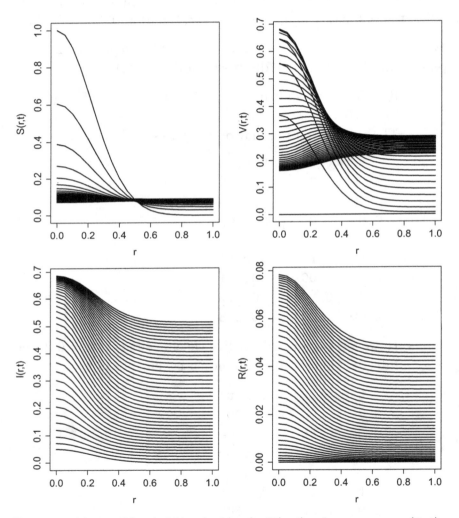

Figure 4.7-1: $S(r,t), V(r,t), I(r,t), R(r,t)$ from eqs. (3.4), $S(r,t=0) = e^{-10r^2}$, $I(r,t=0) = 0.05e^{-10r^2}$, 2D, $\sigma = 0.2$

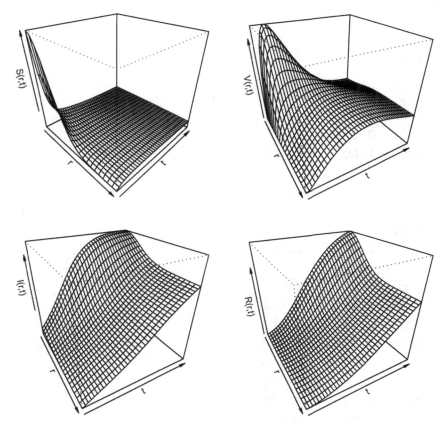

Figure 4.7-2: $S(r,t), V(r,t), I(r,t), R(r,t)$ from eqs. (3.4), $S(r, t = 0) = e^{-10r^2}$, $I(r, t = 0) = 0.05e^{-10r^2}$, 3D, $\sigma = 0.2$

Fig. 4.7-2 indicates the dispersion of the four PDE dependent variables in r with increasing t. The spread of the infected population, $I(r,t)$, is particularly noteworthy.

An increase in the vaccine efficacy, $\sigma = 0.9$ (Listing 4.5), gives the following numerical solution.

[1] 41

[1] 85

```
    t       r       S(r,t)
  0.00    0.00      1.000
  0.00    0.50      0.082
  0.00    1.00      0.000


    t       r       V(r,t)
  0.00    0.00      0.000
  0.00    0.50      0.000
  0.00    1.00      0.000


    t       r       I(r,t)
  0.00    0.00      0.050
  0.00    0.50      0.004
  0.00    1.00      0.000


    t       r       R(r,t)
  0.00    0.00      0.000
  0.00    0.50      0.000
  0.00    1.00      0.000


    t       r       S(r,t)
  1.00    0.00      0.115
  1.00    0.50      0.095
  1.00    1.00      0.093


    t       r       V(r,t)
  1.00    0.00      0.613
  1.00    0.50      0.376
  1.00    1.00      0.350
```

```
  t      r      I(r,t)
1.00   0.00     0.254
1.00   0.50     0.181
1.00   1.00     0.176


  t      r      R(r,t)
1.00   0.00     0.021
1.00   0.50     0.014
1.00   1.00     0.013


  t      r      S(r,t)
2.00   0.00     0.104
2.00   0.50     0.101
2.00   1.00     0.100


  t      r      V(r,t)
2.00   0.00     0.511
2.00   0.50     0.461
2.00   1.00     0.454


  t      r      I(r,t)
2.00   0.00     0.344
2.00   0.50     0.286
2.00   1.00     0.282


  t      r      R(r,t)
2.00   0.00     0.037
2.00   0.50     0.029
2.00   1.00     0.029


ncall =    230
```

Table 4.6: Numerical output from eqs. (3.4), (3.6), (3.7), (3.8), $\sigma = 0.9$, $S(r, t = 0) = e^{-10r^2}$, $I(r, t = 0) = 0.05e^{-10r^2}$

The infected population is reduced.

sigma=0.2, Table 4.5

t	r	I(r,t)
2.00	0.00	0.686
2.00	0.50	0.533
2.00	1.00	0.515

sigma=0.9, Table 4.6

t	r	I(r,t)
2.00	0.00	0.344
2.00	0.50	0.286
2.00	1.00	0.282

The features of the solutions are confirmed in Figs. 4.8.

Fig. 4.8-1 indicates the sharp decrease in the infected population, $I(r,t)$, with the increased vaccine efficacy (compare Figs. 4.7-1 and 4.8-1).

Fig. 4.8-2 indicates the dispersion of the four PDE dependent variables in r with increasing t. Again, the spread of the infected population, $I(r,t)$, is particularly noteworthy.

Table 4.6 indicates that a substantial infected population remains at steady state, e.g., $I(r = 0, t = 2) = 0.344$. This population results from one or more of the positive RHS terms in eqs. (3.3-3), (3.4-3), eps+beta*SI[i]+(1-sigma)*beta*VI[i]. For the next case, $\epsilon = 0.05$ is considered to further reduce $I(r,t)$ (beyond the increased efficacy, $\sigma = 0.9$). The parameters in

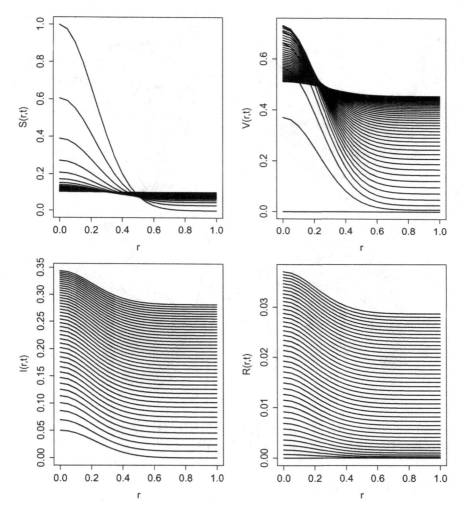

Figure 4.8-1: $S(r,t), V(r,t), I(r,t), R(r,t)$ from eqs. (3.4), $S(r,t=0) = e^{-10r^2}$, $I(r,t=0) = 0.05e^{-10r^2}$, 2D, $\sigma = 0.9$

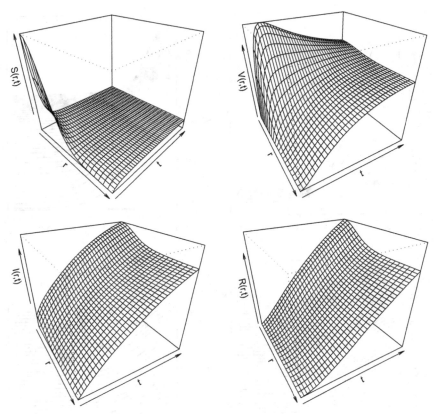

Figure   4.8-2: $S(r,t), V(r,t), I(r,t), R(r,t)$ from   eqs.   (3.4),
$S(r, t = 0) = e^{-10r^2}$, $I(r, t = 0) = 0.05e^{-10r^2}$, 3D, $\sigma = 0.9$

Listings 4.5, 4.7 are

```
#
# Parameters
  alpha=0.25;
  beta=4.5;
  delta=1;
  eps=0.05;
  xi=10;
  omega=1;
```

```
sigma=0.9;
Ds=1.0e-03; Dv=1.0e-03;
Di=1.0e-03; Dr=1.0e-03;
ks=0; kv=0; ki=0; kr=0;
Sb=1; Vb=1; Ib=1; Rb=1;
```

The numerical output (for $\sigma = 0.9, \epsilon = 0.05$) follows.

[1] 41

[1] 85

t	r	S(r,t)
0.00	0.00	1.000
0.00	0.50	0.082
0.00	1.00	0.000

t	r	V(r,t)
0.00	0.00	0.000
0.00	0.50	0.000
0.00	1.00	0.000

t	r	I(r,t)
0.00	0.00	0.050
0.00	0.50	0.004
0.00	1.00	0.000

t	r	R(r,t)
0.00	0.00	0.000
0.00	0.50	0.000
0.00	1.00	0.000

t	r	S(r,t)
1.00	0.00	0.150
1.00	0.50	0.127

1.00	1.00	0.125

t	r	V(r,t)
1.00	0.00	0.748
1.00	0.50	0.495
1.00	1.00	0.467

t	r	I(r,t)
1.00	0.00	0.096
1.00	0.50	0.041
1.00	1.00	0.038

t	r	R(r,t)
1.00	0.00	0.009
1.00	0.50	0.003
1.00	1.00	0.003

t	r	S(r,t)
2.00	0.00	0.146
2.00	0.50	0.142
2.00	1.00	0.141

t	r	V(r,t)
2.00	0.00	0.721
2.00	0.50	0.658
2.00	1.00	0.649

t	r	I(r,t)
2.00	0.00	0.116
2.00	0.50	0.071
2.00	1.00	0.068

t	r	R(r,t)
2.00	0.00	0.013

```
2.00   0.50        0.007
2.00   1.00        0.007

ncall =    230
```

Table 4.7: Numerical output from eqs. (3.4), (3.6), (3.7), (3.8),
$\sigma = 0.9$, $\epsilon = 0.05$, $S(r, t = 0) = e^{-10r^2}$, $I(r, t = 0) = 0.05e^{-10r^2}$

Table 4.7 indicates a further reduction in $I(r, t)$.

```
Table 4.5
sigma=0.2, epsilon=0.25

   t      r      I(r,t)
2.00   0.00      0.686
2.00   0.50      0.533
2.00   1.00      0.515


Table 4.6
sigma=0.9, epsilon=0.25

   t      r      I(r,t)
2.00   0.00      0.344
2.00   0.50      0.286
2.00   1.00      0.282



Table 4.7
sigma=0.9, epsilon=0.05

   t      r      I(r,t)
2.00   0.00      0.116
2.00   0.50      0.071
2.00   1.00      0.068
```

The graphical output in Figs. 4.9 confirms the reduction in $I(r,t)$ (compare Figs. 4.7-1, 4.8-1, 4.9-1).

Fig. 4.9-1 indicates the additional decrease in the infected population, $I(r,t)$, with the decreased ϵ.

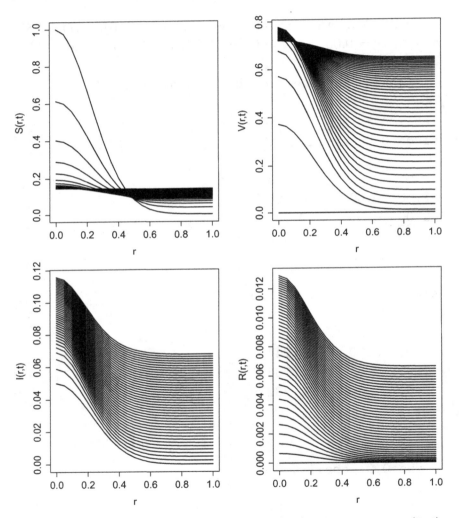

Figure 4.9-1: $S(r,t), V(r,t), I(r,t), R(r,t)$ from eqs. (3.4), $S(r,t=0) = e^{-10r^2}$, $I(r,t=0) = 0.05e^{-10r^2}$, 2D, $\sigma = 0.9$, $\epsilon = 0.05$

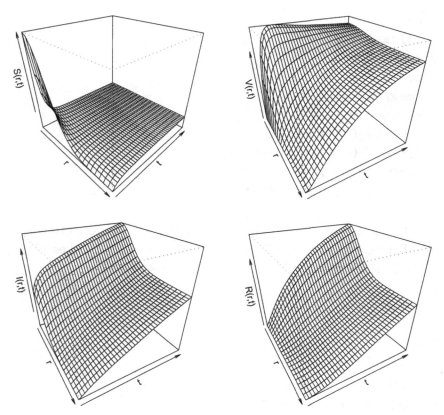

Figure   4.9-2: $S(r,t), V(r,t), I(r,t), R(r,t)$ from   eqs.   (3.4),
$S(r, t = 0) = e^{-10r^2}$, $I(r, t = 0) = 0.05e^{-10r^2}$, 3D, $\sigma = 0.9$,
$\epsilon = 0.05$

The effect of reducing `beta*SI[i]` (RHS of eqs. (3.3-3),
(3.4-3)) is left as an exercise.

As a concluding case, the effect of BCs (3.8) is considered.
Specifically, the parameters in Listings 4.5, 4.7 are

```
#
# Parameters
  alpha=0.25;
```

```
beta=4.5;
delta=1;
eps=0.05;
xi=10;
omega=1;
sigma=0.9;
Ds=1.0e-01; Dv=1.0e-01;
Di=1.0e-01; Dr=1.0e-01;
ks=0; kv=0; ki=1; kr=0;
Sb=1; Vb=1; Ib=1; Rb=1;
```

In particular, `ki=0` is changed to `ki=1` so that nonzero transfer of infecteds across the boundary at $r = r_u = 1$ takes place. That is, the effect of BC (3.8-3) is demonstrated.

```
[1] 41
```

```
[1] 85
```

t	r	S(r,t)
0.00	0.00	1.000
0.00	0.50	0.082
0.00	1.00	0.000

t	r	V(r,t)
0.00	0.00	0.000
0.00	0.50	0.000
0.00	1.00	0.000

t	r	I(r,t)
0.00	0.00	0.050

| 0.00 | 0.50 | 0.004 |
| 0.00 | 1.00 | 0.000 |

t	r	R(r,t)
0.00	0.00	0.000
0.00	0.50	0.000
0.00	1.00	0.000

t	r	S(r,t)
1.00	0.00	0.126
1.00	0.50	0.117
1.00	1.00	0.098

t	r	V(r,t)
1.00	0.00	0.511
1.00	0.50	0.458
1.00	1.00	0.384

t	r	I(r,t)
1.00	0.00	0.107
1.00	0.50	0.237
1.00	1.00	0.814

t	r	R(r,t)
1.00	0.00	0.011
1.00	0.50	0.024
1.00	1.00	0.053

t	r	S(r,t)
2.00	0.00	0.126
2.00	0.50	0.119
2.00	1.00	0.104

t	r	V(r,t)
2.00	0.00	0.561
2.00	0.50	0.521
2.00	1.00	0.463

t	r	I(r,t)
2.00	0.00	0.265
2.00	0.50	0.385
2.00	1.00	0.850

t	r	R(r,t)
2.00	0.00	0.035
2.00	0.50	0.049
2.00	1.00	0.074

ncall =   266

Table 4.8: Numerical output from eqs. (3.4), (3.6), (3.7), (3.8), $\sigma = 0.9$, $\epsilon = 0.05$, $k_I = 1$, $S(r, t = 0) = e^{-10r^2}$, $I(r, t = 0) = 0.05e^{-10r^2}$

The graphical output is in Figs. 4.10.

Fig. 4.10-1 indicates the effect of BC (3.8-3) (at $r = r_u = 1$).

The pronounced effect of BC (3.8-3) is clear by comparing Figs. 4.9 and 4.10. In general, the effect of transfer across the boundary at $r = r_u = 1$ can be demonstrated by varying the transfer coefficients k_S, k_V, k_I, k_R. This is left as an exercise.

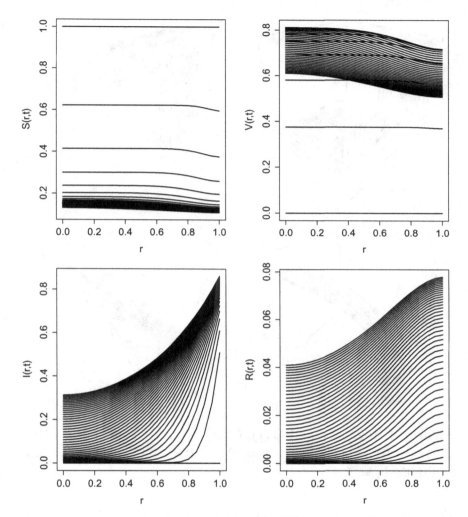

Figure 4.10-1: $S(r,t), V(r,t), I(r,t), R(r,t)$ from eqs. (3.4), $S(r,t=0) = e^{-10r^2}$, $I(r,t=0) = 0.05e^{-10r^2}$, 2D, $\sigma = 0.9$, $\epsilon = 0.05$, $k_I = 1$

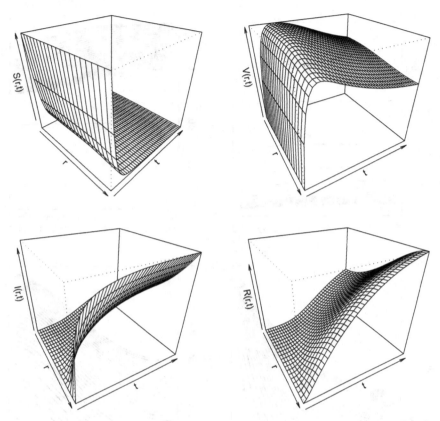

Figure 4.10-2: $S(r,t), V(r,t), I(r,t), R(r,t)$ from eqs. (3.4), $S(r,t=0) = e^{-10r^2}$, $I(r,t=0) = 0.05e^{-10r^2}$, 3D, $\sigma = 0.9$, $\epsilon = 0.05$, $k_I = 1$

(4.3) Summary and conclusions

The implementation of the ODE/PDE SVIR model formulated in Chapter 3 is discussed in this chapter through the following steps:

- The ODE model is implemented in Listings 4.1, 4.2 to demonstrate the solution to eqs. (3.3), (3.5), $S(t)$, $V(t)$,

$I(t)$, $R(t)$, which includes a substantial number of vaccinations and infections with the vaccine efficacy set to a low level, $\sigma = 0.2$

- With the increase in the vaccine efficacy to $\sigma = 0.9$, the number of infections is reduced substantially.
- The derivatives $\dfrac{dS(t)}{dt}, \dfrac{dV(t)}{dt}, \dfrac{dI(t)}{dt}, \dfrac{dR(t)}{dt}$ of eqs. (3.3) are computed and displayed with the code of Listings 4.3, 4.4 to demonstrate the approach to a steady state (the derivatives approach zero).
- The ODE model is extended to include spatial effects in the solution, $S(r, t)$, $V(r, t)$, $I(r, t)$, $R(r, t)$. The resulting PDEs have diffusion in the radial coordinate r, and include diffusivities D_S, D_V, D_I, D_R. The PDEs are second order in r and the two BCs for each PDE are (1) zero Neumann (no flux) at $r = r_l = 0$ (eqs. (3.7)) and (2) Robin at $r = r_u = 1$ (eqs. (3.8)) that equate the diffusion flux to transfer with coefficients k_R, k_V, k_I, k_R with a surrounding region with populations S_b, V_b, I_b, R_b (Listings 4.5, 4.6).
- The solutions with only diffusion in $0 \leq r \leq 1$ are considered for $\sigma = 0.2, 0.9$ by using zero transfer coefficients (Listings 4.5, 4.6). The ICs of eqs. (3.6) are $S(r, t = 0) = 1, V(r, t = 0) = I(r, t = 0) = R(r, t = 0) = 0$, so that the solutions are invariant in r.
- Gaussian ICs give a variation of the solutions in r (Listing 4.7),
- An infusion of infecteds is then added by taking $k_I = 1$ in BC (3.8-3). Adjustment of the diffusivities from 10^{-3} to 10^{-1} gives a clearer indication of the effect of the BC in $I(r = r_u = 1, t)$ which illustrates the interaction of the parameters.

The ODE and PDE models can be studied further with computer-based numerical experimentation using the R routines of Listings 4.1 to 4.7.

References

[1] Schiesser, W.E. (2016), *Method of Lines Analysis in Biomedical Science and Engineering*, John Wiley, Hoboken, NJ, USA

[2] Soetaert, K., J. Cash, and F. Mazzia (2012), *Solving Differential Equations in R*, Springer-Verlag, Heidelberg, Germany.

Appendix A: Function dss004

A listing of function dss004 follows.

```
dss004=function(xl,xu,n,u) {
#
# An extensive set of documentation comments
# detailing the derivation of the following
# fourth order finite differences (FDs) is
# not given here to conserve space.  The
# derivation is detailed in Schiesser, W. E.,
# The Numerical Method of Lines Integration
# of Partial Differential Equations, Academic
# Press, San Diego, 1991.
#
# Preallocate arrays
  ux=rep(0,n);
#
# Grid spacing
  dx=(xu-xl)/(n-1);
#
# 1/(12*dx) for subsequent use
  r12dx=1/(12*dx);
#
# ux vector
#
# Boundaries (x=xl,x=xu)
  ux[1]=r12dx*(-25*u[1]+48*u[  2]-36*u[  3]+
              16*u[  4] -3*u[  5]);
```

161

```
    ux[n]=r12dx*( 25*u[n]-48*u[n-1]+36*u[n-2]-
               16*u[n-3 ] +3*u[n-4]);
#
# dx in from boundaries (x=xl+dx,x=xu-dx)
    ux[  2]=r12dx*(-3*u[1]-10*u[  2]+18*u[  3]-
                6*u[  4]    +u[  5]);
    ux[n-1]=r12dx*( 3*u[n]+10*u[n-1]-18*u[n-2]+
                6*u[n-3]    -u[n-4]);
#
# Interior points (x=xl+2*dx,...,x=xu-2*dx)
    for(i in 3:(n-2)){
      ux[i]=r12dx*(-u[i+2]+8*u[i+1]-
                8*u[i-1]    +u[i-2]);}
#
# All points concluded (x=xl,...,x=xu)
    return(c(ux));
}
```

The input arguments are

        xl   lower boundary value of x

        xu   upper boundary value of x

        n   number of points in the grid in x,
                  including the end points

        u   dependent variable to be differentiated,
                  an n-vector

The output, ux, is an n-vector of numerical values of the first derivative of u.

The finite difference (FD) approximations are a weighted sum of the dependent variable values. For example, at point i

```
#
# Interior points (x=xl+2*dx,...,x=xu-2*dx)
  for(i in 3:(n-2)){
    ux[i]=r12dx*(-u[i+2]+8*u[i+1]-
             8*u[i-1]  +u[i-2]);}
```

The weighting coefficients are -1, 8, 0, -8, 1 at points i-2, i-1, i, i+1, i+2, respectively. These weighting coefficients are antisymmetric (opposite sign) around the center point i because the computed first derivative is of odd order. If the derivative is of even order, the weighting coefficients would be symmetric (same sign) around the center point.

For i=1. the dependent variable at points i=1,2,3,4,5 is used in the FD approximation for ux[1] to remain within the x domain (fictitious points outside the x domain are not used).

```
ux[1]=r12dx*(-25*u[1]+48*u[  2]-36*u[  3]+
            16*u[  4] -3*u[  5]);
```

Similarly, for i=2, points i=1,2,3,4,5 are used in the FD approximation for ux[2] to remain within the x domain (fictitious points outside the x domain are avoided).

```
ux[  2]=r12dx*(-3*u[1]-10*u[  2]+18*u[  3]-
              6*u[  4]  +u[  5]);
```

At the right boundary $x = x_u$, points at i=n,n-1,n-2,n-3,n-4 are used for ux[n],ux[n-1] to avoid points outside the x domain.

In all cases, the FD approximations are fourth order correct in x.

Index